Frontiers in Nano and Micro-Device Design for Applied Nanophotonics, Biophotonics and Nanomedicine

Authored by

A. Guillermo Bracamonte
Instituto de Investigaciones en Físico Química de Córdoba (INFIQC),
Departamento de Química Orgánica,
Facultad de Ciencias Químicas,
Universidad Nacional de Córdoba. Ciudad Universitaria,
5000 Córdoba,
Argentina

&

Departement de chimie and Centre d'optique,
photonique et laser (COPL),
Université Laval, Québec (QC),
Canada

Frontiers in Nano and Micro-Device Design for Applied Nanophotonics, Biophotonics and Nanomedicine

Author: A. Guillermo Bracamonte

ISBN (Online): 978-1-68108-856-3

ISBN (Print): 978-1-68108-857-0

ISBN (Paperback): 978-1-68108-858-7

© 2021, Bentham Books imprint.

Published by Bentham Science Publishers – Sharjah, UAE. All Rights Reserved.

need for a court order if at any point you breach any terms of this License Agreement. In no event will any delay or failure by Bentham Science Publishers in enforcing your compliance with this License Agreement constitute a waiver of any of its rights.

3. You acknowledge that you have read this License Agreement, and agree to be bound by its terms and conditions. To the extent that any other terms and conditions presented on any website of Bentham Science Publishers conflict with, or are inconsistent with, the terms and conditions set out in this License Agreement, you acknowledge that the terms and conditions set out in this License Agreement shall prevail.

Bentham Science Publishers Ltd.
Executive Suite Y - 2
PO Box 7917, Saif Zone
Sharjah, U.A.E.
Email: subscriptions@benthamscience.net

BENTHAM SCIENCE

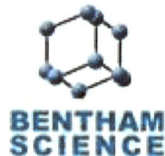

CONTENTS

PREFACE

The aim of this book was to review central concepts of nanoscale by designing and synthesizing different nanomaterials with variable nanoarchitecture, and developing nanodevices and microdevices for nanophotonics, biophotonics and drug delivery applications. Topics ranging from Fluorescence, Plasmonics, Enhanced Plasmonics (EP) to Metal Enhanced Fluorescence (MEF) from colloidal dispersion to single luminescent nanoplatforms and nano-spectroscopy were discussed.

In addition, proof of concepts of microdevices and nanodevices to real applications within genomics, biochemistry, drug delivery and clinical chemistry based on advanced optical detection and imaging were shown, as well as microfluidics, nanofluidics, silica wave-guiding, lasers, nanolasers and photonic circuits for enhanced signal detections.

Latest Nobel-prize awarded developments in Physics and Chemistry on Advanced Laser Instrumentation and applications, Single Molecule detection (SMD) and Biochemistry were also included.

A. Guillermo Bracamonte
Instituto de Investigaciones en Físico Química de Córdoba (INFIQC)
Departamento de Química Orgánica
Facultad de Ciencias Químicas
Universidad Nacional de Córdoba Ciudad Universitaria
5000 Córdoba
Argentina

&

Departement de chimie and Centre d'optique
photonique et laser (COPL)
Université Laval Québec (QC)
Canada

ACKNOWLEDGEMENTS

The author gratefully acknowledge the Département de Chimie and Centre d'Optique, Photonique et Laser (COPL), Québec, Canada, for the postdoctoral research position, the National University of Cordoba (Universidad Nacional de Cordoba, UNC), Argentina, and the National Research Council of Argentina (CONICET) for the research and teaching positions. Special thanks are also due to the Secretary of Science and Technology of UNC (SeCyT), Argentina, for the research grant. Moreover, the author is especially thankful to Professor Denis Boudreau from COPL at Laval University, Québec, Canada, for the long-standing research collaboration in progress as well as to all the Canadian Grants that permit it. Professor Cornelia Bohne, a postdoctoral researcher at the University of Victoria, Victoria in Vancouver Island, British Columbia, Canada, is gratefully acknowledged. Similarly, the author would like to thank Professor Burkhard König from the Institut fur Organische Chemie, Universitat Regensburg, Regensburg, Germany, for the research visit and lecture opportunity provided in his laboratory. Moreover, Professor Nita Sahai from the University of Akron, Institute of Polymer Science and Engineering and NASA Astrobiology Institute, Ohio, United States postdoctoral research position is acknowledged. In addition, the author acknowledges the visit to Professor Jesse Greener Laboratory, in the Département de Chimie forming part of the "http://www.cqmfscience.com/" CQMF (Quebéc Center for Functional Materials) and "http://www.cerma.ulaval.ca/" CERMA (Center for Research on Advanced Materials), at Université Laval, Québec, Canada, and for the discussions held about the design of microfluidic and bioanalytical techniques.

CONSENT FOR PUBLICATION

Not applicable.

CONFLICT OF INTEREST

The author declares no conflict of interest, financial or otherwise.

CHAPTER 1

Introduction to the Basis of Micro- and Nanodevices Design

Abstract: For the design of microdevices and nanodevices, different chemical syntheses need to be controlled to tune the nano- and microscale. Thus, new properties based on the constitution and modification of surface material could be obtained. According to the different material and metamaterial constitutions, variable properties could be developed for targeted applications, including non-classical modes of light, energy transference and smart responsive surfaces. Hence, many designs of lab-on particles, chips and optical circuits, among others, have been discussed from nano- to microscale in nanophotonics, biophotonics, neurophotonics and nanomedicine applications.

Keywords: Chemical synthesis, Development of nanodevices, Microdevices, Nanomaterials, Surface modifications, Tuning of material properties.

1. INTRODUCTION

The control of the nanoscale from atoms and molecules has shown to be the basic concept to scale-up for the development of nanodevices and microdevices. Similarly, the processes and phenomena that took place at shorter nm length and overcame signal loss and interference have allowed showing an impact on the macroscale and real world where it needs to be transferred. Here, multi-disciplinary research interactions have shown the relevance of the control of the nanoscale by methodologies ranging from wet chemistry [1] to nanolithography [1, 2], based on high electron beam [1, 2] and laser applications [1, 2].

In these fields, the design, synthesis and development of new nanomaterials showed a high impact on energy with solar panels and batteries [3, 4], nanomedicine [5] with current advanced point-of-care diagnostics, new treatments from drug delivery [6 - 8], genomic applications [9 - 11], biomedical devices and instrumentation based on the control of surface modification [12, 13], nanotechnological developments such as hybrid Light Emitters Devices (**LEDs**) [14], Organic Light Emitters Devices (**O-LEDs**) [15, 16] and new approaches including Plasmonic Light Emitters Devices (**P-LEDs**) [17], Advanced Optical

Instrumentation such as reduced-size lens based on synthetic nanocrystals [18], semiconductor nanomaterials and conductive nanomaterials with impact on electronics and micro-processors [19], and many other developments where nanoarchitecture control is used as a nanotool and nanoplatform for signal transduction in the frontiers of Quantics and nanoscale [20] to higher levels.

Therefore, from the design and synthesis of tuneable properties based on variable nanoarchitectures for targeted applications, nanodevices could be developed and also incorporated within microdevices (Fig. **1**). The major aspect in the development of these types of nano- and microdevices centers on signal discrimination, enhancement and transduction from the molecular level to the nanoscale and beyond larger surfaces by accurate patterning and excitation.

In the developments and applications mentioned, the study of light interaction and energy with nanomaterial as nanophotonics [21] has proved to be key, having different applications [22].

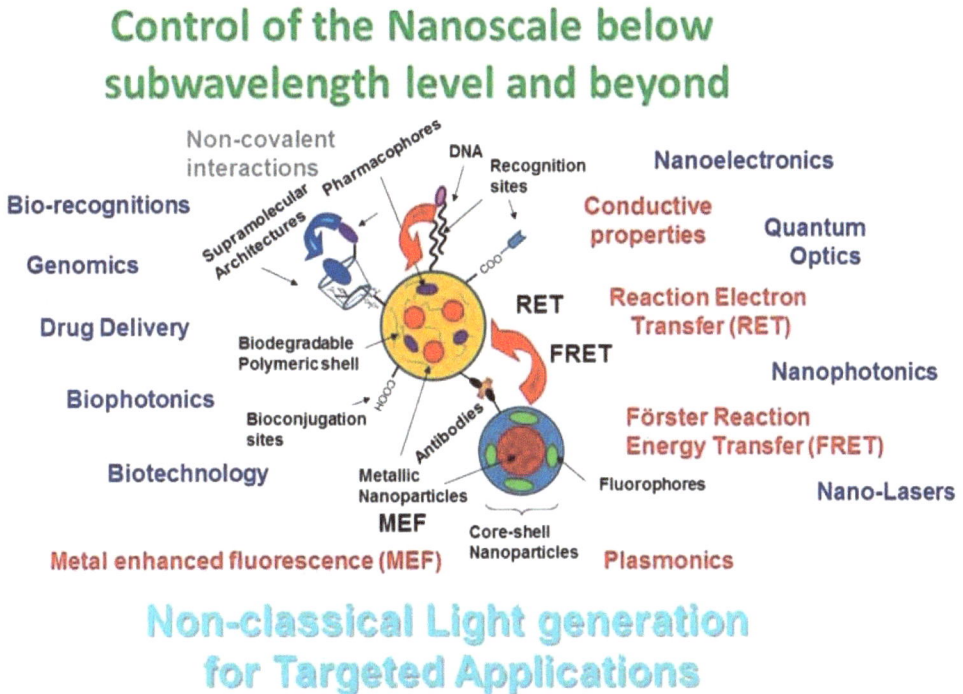

Fig. (1). Scheme of tuneable properties based on variable nanoarchitecture for targeted applications (blue). Type of nanoparticles, chemical modification and physical properties developed (black).

In addition, control of the nanoscale has allowed producing nanofluidic [23] and microfluidic devices [24] where nanomaterials could be confined and combined with variable biostructures for advanced studies. In this way, nano-material characterization has been brought to another level, as well as applications based on detection, tracking and activation of controlled functionalities from individual nano- and microplatforms by advanced optical set-ups coupled to biomaterial and biological samples.

In order to transduce signals from a nanoplatform or from another stimulus within controlled routing, signal waveguiding has been developed from polymeric nanomaterials that allowed controlled and targeted detection and transductions of wavelength signals such as silica waveguides [25] used in the design of microdevices.

Some of these new approaches based on inflow and within conductive materials have been applied to real instrumentation that came into the market and are currently available in research, biochemistry and clinical laboratories [26].

From these levels of control, the design and production of photonic circuits [27] could be mentioned as well, for conventional and no-conventional light transductions, impacting on microdevices, microprocessors and new computers.

Similarly, the nanograting of optical fibers [28] for the development of optosensor has shown studies with high impact and applications in different research fields such as communication, molecular-, bio-sensing and neurophotonics [29].

All the developments just mentioned, related to the control of the nanoscale for nanodevices and microdevices, as well as their incorporation in new set-ups and instrumentation, have enabled advanced biophotonic [30, 31] applications, where accurate targeted light, electronic and physical-chemical process detections have demonstrated to be major challenges to overcome.

Accordingly, studies based on nanoimaging [32] and bioimaging opened up new research fields in Single Molecule Detection (**SMD**) [33], high point-of-care diagnostics and new nanomedicine treatments [34] that reached the genomic level [35].

Probably, these subjects were not interrelated in the early developments. Today, however, from multidisciplinary knowledge, the most advanced applications gained recognition/proved successful in this way.

This chapter discusses the latest developments taking place in nanophotonics, biophotonics, neurophotonics and nanomedicine. In addition, due to the implication of different Plasmonic phenomena in quantum-, nano- and microdevices, we also discussed Enhanced Plasmonics (**EP**) [36], Optical Nanocavities and Resonators (**OR**) [37], Metal Enhanced Fluorescence (**MEF**) [38, 39] and coupled phenomena, as well as Energy Transfer (**ET**) [40] phenomena and Fluorescence Resonance Energy Transfer (**FRET**) [41].

CONCLUDING REMARKS

On the basis of chemical synthesis, it should be noted that material properties could be controlled, as well size, shape, material surface modification and patterning in order to tune materials and properties, from the nanoscale to the microscale, the design and development of targeted nanodevices and microdevices. Multidisciplinary fields are also involved so as to obtain functional devices for nanophotonics, biophotonics and nanomedicine applications.

REFERENCES

[1] T. Ito, and S. Okazaki, "Pushing the limits of lithography", *Nature,* vol. 406, no. 6799, pp. 1027-1031, 2000.
[http://dx.doi.org/10.1038/35023233] [PMID: 10984061]

[2] A. Ródenas, and M. Gu, "Three-dimensional femtosecond laser nanolithography of crystals", *Nature Nanophotonics,* vol. 13, pp. 105-109, 2019.
[http://dx.doi.org/10.1038/s41566-018-0327-9]

[3] J. Wan, T. Song, C. Flox, J. Yang, Q-H. Yang, and X. Han, "Editorial. advanced nanomaterials for energy-related applications", *J. Nanomater,* vol. 2015, no. 564097, pp. 1-2, 2015.

[4] Z.H. Kafafi, R.J. Martín-Palma, A.F. Nogueira, D.M. O'Carroll, J.J. Pietron, I.D.W. Samuel, F. So, N. Tansu, and L. Tsakalakos, "The role of photonics in energy", *Journal of Photonics for Energy,* vol. 050997, no. 5, pp. 1-44, 2015.

[5] B. Pelaz, C. Alexiou, and R.A. Alvarez-Puebla, "Diverse applications of nanomedicine", *ACS Nano,* vol. 11, no. 3, pp. 2313-2381, 2017.
[http://dx.doi.org/10.1021/acsnano.6b06040] [PMID: 28290206]

[6] P. Ghosh, G. Han, M. De, C.K. Kim, and V.M. Rotello, "Gold nanoparticles in delivery applications", *Adv. Drug Deliv. Rev,* vol. 60, no. 11, pp. 1307-1315, 2008.
[http://dx.doi.org/10.1016/j.addr.2008.03.016] [PMID: 18555555]

[7] W. H De Jong, and P. JA Borm, "Drug delivery and nanoparticles: Applications and hazards", *Int. J. Nanomed.,* vol. 3, no. 2, pp. 133-149, 2008.

[8] N.K. Mohtaram, A. Montgomery, and S.M. Willerth, "Biomaterial-based drug delivery systems for the controlled release of neurotrophic factors", *Biomed. Mater,* vol. 8, no. 2, p. 022001, 2013.
[http://dx.doi.org/10.1088/1748-6041/8/2/022001] [PMID: 23385544]

[9] G. Chen, B. Ma, Y. Wang, and S. Gong, "A universal GSH-responsive nanoplatform for the delivery of DNA, mRNA, and Cas9/sgRNA ribonucleoprotein", *ACS Appl. Mater. Interfaces,* vol. 10, no. 22, pp. 18515-18523, 2018.
[http://dx.doi.org/10.1021/acsami.8b03496] [PMID: 29798662]

[10] V.K. Gupta, M.L. Yola, and M.S. Qureshi, "A novel impedimetric biosensor based on graphene oxide/gold nanoplatform for detection of DNA arrays", *Sens. Actuators B Chem,* vol. 188, pp. 1201-121, 2013.
[http://dx.doi.org/10.1016/j.snb.2013.08.034]

[11]   J. Yao, M. Yang, and Y. Duan, "Chemistry, biology, and medicine of fluorescent nanomaterials and related systems: new insights into biosensing, bioimaging, genomics, diagnostics, and therapy", *Chem. Rev,* vol. 114, no. 12, pp. 6130-6178, 2014.
       [http://dx.doi.org/10.1021/cr200359p] [PMID: 24779710]

[12]   A.C.R. Grayson, R.S. Shawgo, A.Y.M. Johnson, N. Flynn, Y. Li, M.J. Cima, and R. Langer, "A BioMEMS review: mems technology for physiologically integrated devices", *Proc. IEEE,* vol. 92, no. 1, pp. 6-21, 2004.
       [http://dx.doi.org/10.1109/JPROC.2003.820534]

[13]   J. Mosinger, K. Lang, and P. Kubát, "Photoactivatable nanostructured surfaces for biomedical applications", *Top. Curr. Chem. (Cham),* vol. 370, pp. 135-168, 2016.
       [http://dx.doi.org/10.1007/978-3-319-22942-3_5] [PMID: 26589508]

[14]   M. Lu, H. Wu, X. Zhang, H. Wang, Y. Hu, V.L. Colvin, Y. Zhang, and W.W. Yu, "Highly flexible Cspbi3 perovskite nanocrystal light-emitting diodes", *ChemNanoMat,* vol. 4, pp. 1-6, 2018.

[15]   D. Volz, "Review of organic light-emitting diodes with thermally activated delayed fluorescence emitters for energy-efficient sustainable light sources and displays", J. Photon. Energy

[16]   B. Xu, W. Wang, X. Zhang, and H. Liu, "Electric bias induced degradation in organic-inorganic hybrid perovskite light-emitting diodes",

[17]   "Nanoscale photonics and optoelectronics", *Lecture Notes in Nanoscale Science and Technology,* vol. 9, pp. 27-46, 2010.

[18]   M-H. Wu, C. Park, and G.M. Whitesides, "Fabrication of arrays of microlenses with controlled profiles using gray-scale microlens projection photolithography", *Langmuir,* vol. 18, no. 24, pp. 9312-9318, 2002.
       [http://dx.doi.org/10.1021/la015735b]

[19]   A. Kamyshny, and S. Magdassi, "Conductive nanomaterials for printed electronics", *Small,* vol. 10, no. 17, pp. 3515-3535, 2014.

[20]   W. Zhou, Y. Y. Zhang, J. Chen, D. Li, J. Zhou, Z. Liu, M. F. Chisholm, S. T. Pantelides, and K. P. Loh, "Dislocation driven growth of two dimensional lateral quantum well super lattices", *Science Advances,* vol. 4, no. eaap9096, pp. 1-7, 2018.

[21]   D.L. Andrews, "Photon-based and classical descriptions in nanophotonics: a review", *J. Nanophotonics,* vol. 081599, no. 8, pp. 1-17, 2014.
       [http://dx.doi.org/10.1117/1.JNP.8.081599]

[22]   N. Rotenberg, and L. Kuipers, "Mapping nanoscale light fields", *Nat. Photonics,* vol. 8, pp. 919-926, 2014.
       [http://dx.doi.org/10.1038/nphoton.2014.285]

[23]   C. Duan, W. Wang, and Q. Xie, "Review article: Fabrication of Nanofluidics devices", *Biomicrofluidics,* vol. 7, no. 026501, pp. 1-41, 2013.

[24]   M. Leester Schadel, T. Lorenz, F. Jurgen, and C. Ritcher, *Fabrication of Microfluidic Devices, Microsystems for Pharmatechnology,* A. Dietzel, Ed., Springer International Publishing: Switzerland, 2016, pp. 23-57.

[25]   M. Kawachi, "Silica waveguides on silicon and their application to integrated-optic components", *Opt. Quantum Electron,* vol. 22, no. 5, pp. 391-416, 1990.
       [http://dx.doi.org/10.1007/BF02113964]

[26]   P. Pearlson, "Austin Suthanthiraraj, S. W. Graves, Fluidics", *Curr. Protoc. Cytom,* vol. 1, no. 2, pp. 1-22, 2013.

[27]   L. Fan, C. L. Zou, R. Cheng, X. Guo, X. Han, Z. Gong, S. Wang, and H. X. Tang, "Superconducting cavity electro optics: A platform for coherent photon conversion between superconducting and photonic circuits", *Sci. Adv.,* vol. 4, no. eaar4994, pp. 1-4, 2018.

[28]   T. Guo, "Fiber grating-assisted surface plasmon resonance for biochemical and electrochemical sensing", *J Lightwave Techn.,* vol. 35, no. 16, pp. 3323-3333, 2017.
[http://dx.doi.org/10.1109/JLT.2016.2590879]

[29]   S. Dufour, and Y. De Koninckc, Optrodes for combined optogenetics and electrophysiology in live animals.*Neurophotonics,* vol. 2,3, no. 031205, pp. 1-14.

[30]   T. Huser, "Nano-biophotonics: new tools for chemical nano-analytics", *Curr. Opin. Chem. Biol.,* vol. 12, no. 5, pp. 497-504, 2008.
[http://dx.doi.org/10.1016/j.cbpa.2008.08.012] [PMID: 18786651]

[31]   E.G. Arthurs, "Perspectives on the future of photonics: the best is yet to come", *Adv. Photonics,* vol. 010501, no. 1, pp. 1-3, 2019.
[http://dx.doi.org/10.1117/1.AP.1.1.010501]

[32]   S. Kawata, "Plasmonics for nanoimaging and nanospectroscopy", *Appl. Spectrosc,* vol. 67, no. 2, pp. 117-125, 2013.
[http://dx.doi.org/10.1366/12-06861] [PMID: 23622428]

[33]   D. Punj, J. de Torres, H. Rigneault, and J. Wenger, "Gold nanoparticles for enhanced single molecule fluorescence analysis at micromolar concentration", *Optics Express,* vol. 27338, no. 21,22, pp. 1-6, 2013.

[34]   J. M. Caster, A. N. Patel, T. Zhang, and A. Wang, "Investigational nanomedicines in 2016: a review of nanotherapeutics currently undergoing clinical trials", *Advanced Review,* vol. 9, pp. 1-9, 2017.

[35]   P. Tebas, D. Stein, W.W. Tang, I. Frank, S.Q. Wang, G. Lee, S.K. Spratt, R.T. Surosky, M.A. Giedlin, G. Nichol, M.C. Holmes, P.D. Gregory, D.G. Ando, M. Kalos, R.G. Collman, G. Binder-Scholl, G. Plesa, W.T. Hwang, B.L. Levine, and C.H. June, "Gene editing of CCR5 in autologous CD4 T cells of persons infected with HIV", *N. Engl. J. Med,* vol. 370, no. 10, pp. 901-910, 2014.
[http://dx.doi.org/10.1056/NEJMoa1300662] [PMID: 24597865]

[36]   B. M. DeVetter, B. E. Bernacki, W. D. Bennett, A. Schemer-Kohrn, and K. J. Alvine, "Multiresonant layered plasmonic films", *J. Nanophoton,* vol. 11,1, no. 016015, pp. 1-8, 2017.

[37]   A. Genç, J. Patarroyo, J. Sancho-Parramon, N.G. Bastús, V. Puntes, and J. Arbiol, "Hollow metal nanostructures for enhanced plasmonics: synthesis, local plasmonic properties and applications, De Gruyer", *Nanophotonics,* pp. 1-21, 2016.

[38]   J.R. Lakowicz, "Radiative decay engineering 5: metal-enhanced fluorescence and plasmon emission", *Anal. Biochem,* vol. 337, no. 2, pp. 171-194, 2005.
[http://dx.doi.org/10.1016/j.ab.2004.11.026] [PMID: 15691498]

[39]   D. Darvill, A. Centeno, and F. Xie, "Plasmonic fluorescence enhancement by metal nanostructures: shaping the future of bionanotechnology", *Phys. Chem. Chem. Phys,* vol. 15, no. 38, pp. 15709-15726, 2013.
[http://dx.doi.org/10.1039/c3cp50415h] [PMID: 23579473]

[40]   S. Hammes-Schiffer, "Proton-coupled electron transfer: moving together and charging forward", *J. Am. Chem. Soc,* vol. 137, no. 28, pp. 8860-8871, 2015.
[http://dx.doi.org/10.1021/jacs.5b04087] [PMID: 26110700]

[41]   H. Dacres, J. Wang, M.M. Dumancic, and S.C. Trowell, "Experimental determination of the forster distance for two commonly used bioluminescent resonance energy transfer pairs", *Anal. Chem,* vol. 82, no. 1, pp. 432-435, 2010.
[http://dx.doi.org/10.1021/ac9022956] [PMID: 19957970]

CHAPTER 2

Control of the Nanoscale Concepts

Abstract: The basis of the nanoscale control was shown and discussed according to different methods of synthesis applying accurate controlled organized media conditions depending on the required size and shape of nanostructures. The importance of chemical surface modification that determined inter-nanoparticle interactions was also underlined, in addition to the final properties based on the nanomaterial constitution.

Keywords: Control of the nanoscale, Chemical surface modification, Effect of size and shape, Hamaker constant, Inter-nanoparticle interactions, Nanomaterial properties, Plasmonics, Synthesis of nanomaterials.

1. CONTROL OF NANOPARTICLE SIZE

Accurate size control at the nanoscale dimension still represents a major challenge due to its implication in tuning the properties of the nanomaterial as well as in its targeted functionality.

The synthetic methodology used depends on the nanomaterial needed and the targeted application. Within colloidal dispersion, variable degrees of dispersibility could be obtained, from dimmers, trimmers and tetramers to higher nanoaggregates, according to the chemical surface interaction. Hence, different properties could be obtained depending on the nanomaterial. In addition, the size of a nanomaterial, along with a given property, determines the success of the targeted application.

For drug delivery applications, the use of biocompatible nanomaterials is required. For this reason, not any nanomaterial could be used, and studies should be developed *in vitro* and *in vivo*. Still, variable levels of immune response could be detected against synthetic material. Moreover, size could determine incorporation by cells, cargo drug loading and release. Larger cargo nanoparticles could load higher concentrations than smaller ones; yet, depending on the kind of administration, different results could be found. For injectable applications, sizes below 100.0 nm showed to be the best dimensions, while for oral administration, where the nanoparticle should cross different barriers, higher dimensions could be used. However, at this point, the importance of size [1] for membrane interaction [2] and surface charge in cellular uptake pathway [3] should be highlighted.

For biosensing, according to the application, the nanoscale could vary. For example, molecular detection based on different detection techniques reduced sizes were required, even close to quantum sizes. Instead, for biostructure detection based on targeted nanolabelling, intermediate sizes could be used [4]. Similarly, for Imaging applications such as nanoimaging and bioimaging based on fluorescence, the size of nanoparticles showed variable intensities, leading to different nanoresolutions. This basic concept from optics was even applied to enhanced resolution based on a switch on/off fluorescence of individual molecules, honoured with a Nobel Prize in Chemistry 2014 shared by Germany and USA [5].

In nanoelectronics, catalysis and electrochemistry, nanomaterial is a key component, having the effect of reduced nanoparticle size and larger surface area to volume ratios that produce increased catalysis and electrochemical response [6].

For in flow methodologies, lab-on chips and lab-on particles, the size of nanoparticles showed to be a central control parameter depending on their applications. For instance, the capability of the design of micro- to nanochannels confines dimensions at different scales and allows passing through targeted sizes [7]. Similarly, in lab-on chips [8] and lab-on particle [9], the size of the nanoparticle, such as nanoplatform for molecular and biostructure detection should be controlled as well. It is particularly interesting to determine, per nanoparticle, how many molecules are deposed, and control their sizes to tune the detection signal of biostructures [10]. Thus, the importance of size control to tune properties for targeted applications where external factors such as media constraints should be stressed.

2. SYNTHESIS, TYPE OF REACTIONS AND NANOMATERIALS IN ORGANIZED MEDIA

For the synthesis and development of the different nanomaterials reported in the literature, there are many types of reactions in the presence of different organized media within colloidal dispersion. Even if this section has not been conceived for detailed procedures, it has been interesting in order to show the most common types of reactions applied over the last years, in addition to highlighting the influence of non-covalent interactions within reaction media to control size, shape, the stability of the colloidal dispersion, and nanopatterns [11 - 13].

Besides wet chemistry methodologies, we should mention nanolithography techniques with high-energy electron beams and lasers on modified surfaces for accurate nanoarchitecture patterning [14]. In colloidal dispersion, the different types of reactions could be classified according to nanomaterial properties. For example, in inorganic nanoparticles such as cooper [15], silver [16] and gold [17], nanoparticles showed different syntheses by reduction reactions with varying strength of reducing agents [18]. Therefore, based on the molar ratios of reactants and the strength of reducing agents, the size of the nanoparticles was controlled. Moreover, for magnetic nanoparticles based on iron, different oxidation/reduction reactions were used with special care in the application of passivating agents for the stabilization of these nanoparticles [19]. Here, we should highlight the importance of the capping agents in the nanoaggregation properties based on their different inter-nanoparticle interactions according to the nanomaterials used. It should also be noted that not all of the most well-known nanoparticles formed by the most commonly known nanomaterials showed the same dispersibility and homogeneity in shape distribution.

Hence, the synthesis is still a considerable challenge for improved colloidal stability and controlled size and shape. In particular, for shape control, different organized media were used to control from the nucleation of a few atoms to the spatial 3D crystal growth. For example, spherical gold nanoparticles were reported with the application of citrate [20] and borohydride [21], as soft and strong reducing agents, respectively. However, in the presence of cetyl trimethyl ammonium bromide (CTAB), longitudinal nanoparticle growth was observed, obtaining nano-rods [22].

Another important variable for control depending on the nanomaterial was the use of controlled atmospheres for the synthesis of nanoparticles that showed higher tendencies to get oxidized, if their size, shape, and property could not be drastically changed, as in nanoparticles of aluminium [23] and indium [24] oxides.

Moreover, within inorganic nanoparticles, silica nanoparticles based on their particular intrinsic excellent properties, including dielectric material and optical transparent characteristics, allowed a considerable/significant number of developments, from nanoplatforms in colloidal dispersion to microdevices based on film deposition and surface modification in numerous research areas such as silica nanophotonics and photovoltaics.

The synthesis of silica nanoparticles was reported by the Sol.-gel Störber method [25] based on an acid/basic catalyzed reaction for condensation of different organosilane monomers (Fig. **1**). These nanoparticles showed high dispersibility in polar media due to their hydroxylated surface, also allowing their chemical surface modification.

Fig. (1). Schematic mechanism of condensation of Silanes *via* acid or base catalysis **A)** With retention of configuration. **B)** With siloxane bond hydrolysis [25].

For organic nanoparticles, polymeric materials based on different types of reaction of polymerization and co-polymerization in the presence of variable monomers allowed obtaining tuneable properties of polymeric Nanomaterials. For example, biodegradable nanoparticles could be obtained by ester condensations in the presence of different organic solvent ratios. Thus, the most commonly known biodegradable nanoparticles, such as polyglycolic, lactic and malic acids, were obtained by multiple-solvent diffusion methodology, inducing monomer condensation by solvent evaporation [26]. Moreover, other polymeric nano-materials should be mentioned from the combination of different molecular properties to monomers and functional polymeric materials such as flexible [27], stretchable organic [28], conductive [29] and wearable organic polymers [30].

In addition, the application of supramolecular interactions as non-covalent linkers for supra nanoparticle architectures aroused interest in many research areas [31]. Similarly, DNA origamis, based on stable non-covalent interactions, showed to be advanced materials with potential application from biomaterial fields [32] to encryption of information and digital information storage [33].

3. EFFECT OF SIZE AND INTERACTION

Control of nanoparticle size showed to be a key factor in nanoaggregation properties. Size as a main variable, irrespective of chemical surfaces, could tune the size of aggregates in colloidal dispersion and over surface deposition.

The nanoaggregation of silver and gold nanoparticles was correlated with Hamaker constants [34]. These constants were based on non-covalent interaction of nanoparticles such as Vander der Walls interactions. Consequently, higher nanoaggregates were measured in the presence of smaller nanoparticles. Sizes smaller than 50.0 nm correlated with higher Hamaker constants and sizes of aggregates. Moreover, these interactions showed dependency on the temperature of colloidal dispersions [35] and counter-ions [36] that governed/determined/ influenced the motion and dynamics of nanoparticles. It should be noted that Hamaker constants could be determined for inorganic [37] and organic nanoparticles by different spectroscopical methodologies [38].

However, chemical surface modification was another key factor for control in order to tune interactions, nanopatterning and biocompatibilities based on different types of non-covalent interactions and development of surface charges [39]. These properties could be measured, for instance, by Dynamic Light Scattering (DLS) [40] techniques, Raman spectroscopy from modification of band absorption of interacting functional groups [41], and surface charge potential developed from these functional chemical groups as well, by Z-Potential measurements [42].

In addition, it should be noted that from their inter-nanoparticle interaction from variable nanomaterial compositions, different physical and chemical nanomaterial properties could be developed. Within these modified properties, modification of high energy electromagnetic fields [43], Quantum confinement [44], magnetic properties [45], thermal conduction properties [46], enhanced catalysis [47] and generation of non-classical light [48] have been reported. Thus, control of size and nanoaggregation is important due to accuracy at the nanoscale but also to their final nanomaterial properties.

4. CHEMICAL SURFACE MODIFICATION

The chemical surface modification of nanostructures should be specially considered due to their internanoparticle interactions and chemical group functionalization, covalent and non-covalent linking of molecules and biostructures, stabilization of surfaces in different media [49], deposition and generation of nanostructured nanopatterns [50], tuning of targeted surface functionalities [51 - 54], biocompatibilization [55] and bioconjugation [56, 57].

Chemical surface modification could be achieved by different chemical reactions produced in colloidal dispersion from which each individual nanoparticle surface interacts with reagents. Hence, chemical reactions are produced along with chemical modification over individual nanoplatforms [58]. Then these nanoplatforms could be applied to further modifications [59] depending on targeted functionalization [60].

5. PLASMONICS IN THE NEAR FIELD AND FRONTIERS IN THE QUANTUM REGIME

Controlling the nanoscale, the dimension related to molecular spacer lengths and quantum confinements could be attained. Below 5.0 nm, new electronic states were reported, showing new electronic properties [61]. These sizes were achieved by synthetic methodologies in colloidal dispersion of semiconductor materials such as quantum dots [62, 63]. It was also possible to achieve metallic nanoparticles sizes close to the Quantum regime by a reduction reaction [64].

At these sizes the generation of quantized photons was reported on demand from an accurate excitation, for example photonic quantum teleportation by fiber coupling [65]. Moreover, in advanced quantum applications, it should not only be able to generate new non-classical states of light, but also control single photon topological states in an integrated photonic circuit to improve the performance and scalability of new quantum dot technologies [66]. In addition, quantum optics showed increased importance in physics and engineering of electronic components based on quantum electronic dynamics, from where lasing modes have demonstrated relevance for low threshold lasers and quantum information processing [67]. At this nanoscale, we should highlight the importance and impact of the application of nanolithography techniques for future quantum computation and networks that require scalable monolithic circuits, incorporating various advanced functionalities in a single physical substrate [68].

In addition, for application to colloidal dispersions based on luminescent quantum dots, quantum nanoplatforms for molecular sensing [69] and biolabelling [70] were reported. Due to their versatility in colloidal dispersion, many strategies have been developed for improved biocompatibility for assays *in vivo* and in-vitro [71] as well.

Similarly, at short distances from the metallic surface known as the near field, the generation of high energy electromagnetic fields named as Plasmons was reported. These electromagnetic fields should be produced by an appropriate laser excitation of the electron of the nanosurfaces. Then, depending on the intrinsic electronic properties of the nanomaterial excited, variable absorption wavelengths could be recorded as well as high energy plasmonic emissions. These plasmonic lasing modes [72] were also applied for enhanced low threshold nanolaser fabrications [73] and plasmonic signal waveguiding [74], resonant-plasmonic waveguiding [75] and enhanced nanophotonic microcircuits [76] could be designed from the right tuning of plasmonic nanocomposites [77].

CONCLUDING REMARKS

The control of the size and shape of the nanomaterial defined interactions and final nanomaterial properties, whereas chemical surface modifications allowed targeted functionalities to interact with the surrounding media. Moreover, from these media sensing, different signal transductions could be recorded, generating the targeted applications according to the different constitutive parts of the nanomaterials that should accurately be placed within the nanoscale.

REFERENCES

[1]   M. Moddaresi, M.B. Brown, Y. Zhao, S. Tamburic, and S.A. Jones, "The role of vehicle-nanoparticle interactions in topical drug delivery", *Int. J. Pharm.,* vol. 400, no. 1-2, pp. 176-182, 2010.
[http://dx.doi.org/10.1016/j.ijpharm.2010.08.012] [PMID: 20727392]

[2]   S. Wang, J. Li, Z. Zhou, S. Zhou, and Z. Hu, "Micro/nano-scales direct cell behavior on biomaterial surfaces", *Molecules,* vol. 24, no. 1, pp. 1-13, 2018.
[http://dx.doi.org/10.3390/molecules24010075] [PMID: 30587800]

[3]   E. Fröhlich, "The role of surface charge in cellular uptake and cytotoxicity of medical nanoparticles", *Int. J. Nanomedicine,* vol. 7, pp. 5577-5591, 2012.
[http://dx.doi.org/10.2147/IJN.S36111] [PMID: 23144561]

[4]   O. Betzer, R. Meir, T. Dreifuss, K. Shamalov, M. Motiei, A. Shwartz, K. Baranes, C.J. Cohen, N. Shraga-Heled, G. Yadid, and R. Popovtzer, "*In-vitro* Optimization of Nanoparticle-Cell Labeling Protocols for *In-vivo* Cell Tracking Applications"., *Nature,* vol. 5, no. 15400, pp. 1-11, 2015.

[5]   E. Betzig, S.W. Hell, and W.E. Moerner, *The Nobel Prize in Chemistry 2014, For the Development of a Super Resolved Fluorescence Microscopy* Press Release from The Royal Swedish Academy of Sciences, 2014.

[6]   M. Samim, N. K. Kaushik, and A. Maitra, "Effect of size of copper nanoparticles on its catalytic behaviour in Ullman reaction", *Bull. Mater. Sci,* vol. 5, no. 2007, pp. 535-540, 2007.

[7]   C. Duan, W. Wang, and Q. Xie, "Review article: Fabrication of nanofluidic devices", *Biomicrofluidics,* vol. 7, no. 2, p. 26501, 2013.

[http://dx.doi.org/10.1063/1.4794973] [PMID: 23573176]

[8]   A.S. Paterson, B. Raja, V. Mandadi, B. Townsend, M. Lee, A. Buell, B. Vu, J. Brgoch, and R.C. Willson, "A low-cost smartphone-based platform for highly sensitive point-of-care testing with persistent luminescent phosphors", *Lab Chip*, vol. 17, no. 6, pp. 1051-1059, 2017.
[http://dx.doi.org/10.1039/C6LC01167E] [PMID: 28154873]

[9]   A. Burns, H. Ow, and U. Wiesner, "Fluorescent core-shell silica nanoparticles: towards "Lab on a Particle" architectures for nanobiotechnology", *Chem. Soc. Rev.*, vol. 35, no. 11, pp. 1028-1042, 2006.
[http://dx.doi.org/10.1039/B600562B] [PMID: 17057833]

[10]   A.V. Veglia, and A.G. Bracamonte, "β-Cyclodextrin grafted gold nanoparticles with short molecular spacers applied for nanosensors based on plasmonic effects", *Microchem. J.*, vol. 148, pp. 277-284, 2019.
[http://dx.doi.org/10.1016/j.microc.2019.04.066]

[11]   C.J. Murphy, T.K. Sau, A.M. Gole, C.J. Orendorff, J. Gao, L. Gou, S.E. Hunyadi, and T. Li, "Anisotropic metal nanoparticles: Synthesis, assembly, and optical applications", *J. Phys. Chem. B,* vol. 109, no. 29, pp. 13857-13870, 2005.
[http://dx.doi.org/10.1021/jp0516846] [PMID: 16852739]

[12]   S. Wolf, and C. Feldmann, "Microemulsions: options to expand the synthesis of inorganic nanoparticles", *Angew. Chem. Int. Ed. Engl.*, vol. 55, no. 51, pp. 15728-15752, 2016.
[http://dx.doi.org/10.1002/anie.201604263] [PMID: 27862742]

[13]   Z. Li, Y. Wang, G. Tian, P. Li, L. Zhao, F. Zhang, J. Yao, H. Fan, X. Song, D. Chen, Z. Fan, M. Qin, M. Zeng, Z. Zhang, X. Lu, S. Hu, C. Lei, Q. Zhu, J. Li, X. Gao, and J-M. Liu, "High-density array of ferroelectric nanodots with robust and reversibly switchable topological domain states", *Sci. Adv.*, vol. 3, no. 8, 2017.e1700919
[http://dx.doi.org/10.1126/sciadv.1700919] [PMID: 28835925]

[14]   A. Pimpin, and W. Srituravanich, "Review on micro and nanolithography techniques and their applications", *Eng. J. (N.Y.),* vol. 16, no. 1, pp. 37-55, 2011.

[15]   Q. Zhang, Z. Yang, B. Ding, X. Lan, and Y. Guo, "Preparation of copper nanoparticles by chemical reduction method using potassium borohydride", *Trans. Nonferrous Met. Soc. China*, vol. 20, pp. s240-s244, 2010.
[http://dx.doi.org/10.1016/S1003-6326(10)60047-7]

[16]   P.J. Rivero, J. Goicoechea, A. Urrutia, and F.J. Arregui, "Effect of both protective and reducing agents in the synthesis of multicolor silver nanoparticles", *Nanoscale Res. Lett.*, vol. 8, no. 1, p. 101, 2013.
[http://dx.doi.org/10.1186/1556-276X-8-101] [PMID: 23432942]

[17]   K. Rahme, and J.D. Holmes, *Gold Nanoparticles: Synthesis, Characterization, and Bioconjugation, Dekker Encyclopedia of Nanoscience and Nanotechnology.* 3rd ed. Taylor and Francis, 2015, pp. 1-11.

[18]   I. Capek, "Nobel Metal Nanoparticles. Preparation, composite Nanostructures", *Biodecoration and Collective Properties, XVII,* vol. 554, pp. 125-210, 2017.

[19]   A.G. Nene, M. Takahashi, and P.R. Somani, "Fe3O4 and Fe Nanoparticles by Chemical Reduction of Fe(acac)3 by Ascorbic Acid: Role of Water", *World Journal of Nano Science and Engineering,* vol. 6, pp. 20-28, 2016.
[http://dx.doi.org/10.4236/wjnse.2016.61002]

[20]   B.V. Enustund, and J. Turkevich, "Coagulation of Colloidal gold", *J. Am. Chem. Soc.*, vol. 85, no. 21, pp. 3317-3328, 1963.
[http://dx.doi.org/10.1021/ja00904a001]

[21]   E.G. Wrigglesworth, and J.H. Johnston, "The use of dual reductant in gold nanoparticle syntheses", *RSC Advances,* vol. 7, pp. 45757-45762, 2017.
[http://dx.doi.org/10.1039/C7RA07724F]

[22]   A.K. Samal, T.S. Sreeprasad, and T. Pradeep, "Investigation of the role of NaBH4 in the chemical

synthesis of gold nanorods", *J. Nanopart. Res.,* vol. 12, pp. 1777-1786, 2010.
[http://dx.doi.org/10.1007/s11051-009-9733-8]

[23] K. A. S. Fernando, M. J. Smith, B. A. Harruff, W. K. Lewis, E. A. Guliants, and C. E. Bunker, "Sonochemically Assisted Thermal Decomposition of Alane N,N-Dimethylethylamine with Titanium (IV) Isopropoxide in the Presence of Oleic Acid to Yield Air-Stable and Size-Selective Aluminum Core-Shell Nanoparticles", *J. Phys. Chem,* vol. 113, no. 2, pp. 500-503, 2009.
[http://dx.doi.org/10.1021/jp809295e] [PMID: jp809295e]

[24] C. Kind, and C. Feldmann, "One-pot synthesis of in0 nanoparticles with tuned particle size and high oxidation stability", *Chem. Mater.,* vol. 23, pp. 4982-4987, 2011.
[http://dx.doi.org/10.1021/cm202256t]

[25] C.J. Brinker, and G.W. Scherer, *Sol-Gel Science. The Physics and Chemistry of Sol-Gel Processing, United Kingdom Edition published by Academic Press.* Elsevier, 1990.

[26] X. Y. Jiang, C. S. Zhou, and K. W. Tang, *Preparation of PLA and PLGA nanoparticles by binary organic solvent diffusion method.*
[http://dx.doi.org/10.1016/s0378-5173(99)00187-8] [PMID: 10502620]

[27] J. Kenry, "Chuan Yeo, C. Teck Lim, Emerging flexible and wearable physical sensing platforms for healthcare and biomedical applications, Microsystems & Nanoengineering", *Nature,* vol. 2, no. 16043, pp. 1-18, 2016.

[28] Y. Lee, J. Young Oh, W. Xu, O. Kim, T. Roy Kim, J. Kang, Y. Kim, D. Son, J. B.-H. Tok, M. Jeong Park, Z. Bao, and T.-W. Lee, "Stretchable organic optoelectronic sensorimotor synapse", *Sci. Adv.,* vol. 4, no. 11, pp. 1-9, 2018.
[http://dx.doi.org/10.1126/sciadv.aat7387]

[29] A. Kamyshny, and S. Magdassi, *Conductive Nanomaterials for Printed Electronics, small,* vol. 10, no. 17, pp. 3515-3535, 2014.

[30] A.K. Bansal, S. Hou, O. Kulyk, E.M. Bowman, and I.D.W. Samuel, "Wearable organic optoelectronic sensors for medicine", *Adv. Mater.,* vol. 27, no. 46, pp. 7638-7644, 2015.
[http://dx.doi.org/10.1002/adma.201403560] [PMID: 25488890]

[31] J. W. Steed, and P. A. Gale, *Supramolecular Chemistry: From Molecules to Nanomaterials,,* vol. 8, pp. 1-4014, 2012.

[32] J. Zhang, T. Lan, and Y. Lu, "Molecular engineering of functional nucleic acid nanomaterials toward in vivo applications", *Adv. Healthc. Mater.,* vol. 8, no. 6, 2019.e1801158
[http://dx.doi.org/10.1002/adhm.201801158] [PMID: 30725526]

[33] G.M. Church, Y. Gao, and S. Kosuri, "Next-generation digital information storage in DNA", *Science,* vol. 337, no. 6102, pp. 1628-1629, 2012.
[http://dx.doi.org/10.1126/science.1226355] [PMID: 22903519]

[34] "P. Pin c h u k; K. Jia n g, Size-dependent Hamaker constants for silver and gold nanoparticles, P r o c. S P I E 9549", *Physical Chemistry of Interfaces and Nanomaterials XIV,* vol. 95491J, pp. 1-3, 2015.

[35] "K Jiang1, P Pinchuk, Temperature and size-dependent Hamaker constants for metal nanoparticles", *Nanotechnology,* vol. 27, no. 345710, pp. 1-9, 2016.

[36] C. Gutsche, U.F. Keyser, K. Kegler, F. Kremer, and P. Linse, "Forces between single pairs of charged colloids in aqueous salt solutions", *Phys. Rev. E Stat. Nonlin. Soft Matter Phys.,* vol. 76, no. 3 Pt 1, 2007.031403
[http://dx.doi.org/10.1103/PhysRevE.76.031403] [PMID: 17930243]

[37] L. Bergstr6m, "Hamaker constants of inorganic materials", *Adv. Colloid Interface Sci.,* vol. 70, pp. 125-169, 1997.
[http://dx.doi.org/10.1016/S0001-8686(97)00003-1]

[38] S. Noskov, C. Scherer, and M. Maskos, "Determination of Hamaker constants of polymeric

nanoparticles in organic solvents by asymmetrical flow field-flow fractionation", *J. Chromatogr. A,* vol. 1274, pp. 151-158, 2013.
[http://dx.doi.org/10.1016/j.chroma.2012.12.001] [PMID: 23273632]

[39]   H. Jans, X. Liu, L. Austin, G. Maes, and Q. Huo, "Dynamic light scattering as a powerful tool for gold nanoparticle bioconjugation and biomolecular binding studies", *Anal. Chem.,* vol. 81, no. 22, pp. 9425-9432, 2009.
[http://dx.doi.org/10.1021/ac901822w] [PMID: 19803497]

[40]   S.K. Brar, and M. Verma, "Measurement of nanoparticles by light-scattering techniques", *Trends Analyt. Chem.,* vol. 30, no. 1, pp. 4-17, 2011.
[http://dx.doi.org/10.1016/j.trac.2010.08.008]

[41]   A.F. Jaramillo, R. Baez-Cruza, L.F. Montoyaa, C. Medinam, E. Pérez-Tijerinad, F. Salazare, D. Rojasa, and M.F. Melendreza, "Estimation of the surface interaction mechanism of ZnO nanoparticles modified with organosilane groups by Raman Spectroscopy", *Ceram. Int.,* vol. 43, pp. 11838-11847, 2017.
[http://dx.doi.org/10.1016/j.ceramint.2017.06.027]

[42]   Y. Yu, P.M. Bacherikov, and O.B. Lytvyn, "Doroshkevich, Surface potential of meso-dimensional ZnS:Mn particles obtained using SHS method", *J. Nanopart. Res.,* vol. 20, no. 316, pp. 1-6, 2018.

[43]   E. Hao, and G.C. Schatz, "Electromagnetic fields around silver nanoparticles and dimers", *J. Chem. Phys.,* vol. 120, no. 1, pp. 357-366, 2004.
[http://dx.doi.org/10.1063/1.1629280] [PMID: 15267296]

[44]   H. Gross, J. M. Hamm, T. Tufarelli, O. Hess, and B. Hecht, "Near field strong coupling of single quantum dots", *Science Advances,* vol. 4, pp. 1-8, 2018.
[PMID: eaar4906]

[45]   H. Kim, A. Palacio Morales, T. Posske, L. Rozsa, K. Palotas, L. Szunyogh, M. Thorwart, and R. Wiesendanger, "", *Science Advances,* vol. 4, p. 1, 2018.
[PMID: eaar5251]

[46]   N. Tsujii, A. Nishide, J. Hayakawa, and T. Mori, "Observation of Enhnaced thermopower due to spin fluctuation in weak itinerant ferromagnet", *Science Advances,* vol. 5, pp. 1-8, 2019.
[PMID: eaat5935]

[47]   B. Munkhbat, M. Wersall, D. G. Baranov, T. J. Antosiewicz, and T. Shegai, "Suppression of photo oxidation of organic chromophores by strong coupling to plasmonic nanoantennas", *Science Advances,* vol. 4, no. eaas9552, pp. 1-11, 2018.

[48]   N. Rotenberg, and L. Kuipers, "Mapping nanoscale light fields", *Nat. Photonics,* vol. 8, pp. 919-926, 2014.
[http://dx.doi.org/10.1038/nphoton.2014.285]

[49]   H. Chen, L. Zhao, D. Chen, and W. Hu, "Stabilization of gold nanoparticles on glass surface with polydopamine thin film for reliable LSPR sensing", *J. Colloid Interface Sci.,* vol. 460, pp. 258-263, 2015.
[http://dx.doi.org/10.1016/j.jcis.2015.08.075] [PMID: 26343978]

[50]   Y. Liu, W. Xiong, L. J. Jiang, Y. S. Zhou, and Y. F. Lu, "Precise 3D printing of micro/nanostructures using highly conductive carbon nanotube-thiolacrylate composites", *Proc. SPIE 9738, Laser 3D Manufacturing III,* vol. , no. , pp. 1-2, 2016.
[http://dx.doi.org/10.4061/2011/973808] [PMID: 973808]

[51]   M. Corredor, D. Carbajo, C. Domingo, Y. Pérez, J. Bujons, A. Messeguer, and I. Alfonso, "Dynamic covalent identification of an efficient heparin ligand", *Angew. Chem. Int. Ed. Engl.,* vol. 57, no. 37, pp. 11973-11977, 2018.
[http://dx.doi.org/10.1002/anie.201806770] [PMID: 29998599]

[52]   A. Müller, and B. König, "Vesicular aptasensor for the detection of thrombin", *Chem. Commun.*

(Camb.), vol. 50, no. 84, pp. 12665-12668, 2014.
[http://dx.doi.org/10.1039/C4CC05221H] [PMID: 25205174]

[53]   D. Schumacher, J. Helma, A.F.L. Schneider, H. Leonhardt, and C.P.R. Hackenberger, "Nanobodies: Chemical Functionalization Strategies and Intracellular Applications", *Angew. Chem. Int. Ed. Engl.,* vol. 57, no. 9, pp. 2314-2333, 2018.
[http://dx.doi.org/10.1002/anie.201708459] [PMID: 28913971]

[54]   Y. Chen, J.M. Cordero, H. Wang, D. Franke, O.B. Achorn, F.S. Freyria, I. Coropceanu, H. Wei, O. Chen, D.J. Mooney, and M.G. Bawendi, "A ligand system for the flexible functionalization of quantum dots via click chemistry", *Angew. Chem. Int. Ed. Engl.,* vol. 57, no. 17, pp. 4652-4656, 2018.
[http://dx.doi.org/10.1002/anie.201801113] [PMID: 29479792]

[55]   W.H. Tse, L. Gyenis, D.W. Litchfield, and J. Zhang, "Cellular interaction influenced by surface modification strategies of gelatin-based nanoparticles", *J. Biomater. Appl.,* vol. 31, no. 7, pp. 1087-1096, 2017.
[http://dx.doi.org/10.1177/0885328216684651] [PMID: 28178901]

[56]   J. Kalia, and R.T. Raines, "Advances in Bioconjugation", *Curr. Org. Chem.,* vol. 14, no. 2, pp. 138-147, 2010.
[http://dx.doi.org/10.2174/138527210790069839] [PMID: 20622973]

[57]   G.T. Hermanson, *Bioconjugate Techniques* 2nd Elsevier. , 2008.

[58]   X. Hai, X. Lin, X. Chen, and J. Wang, "Highly selective and sensitive detection of cysteine with a graphene quantum dots-gold nanoparticles based core-shell nanosensor", *Sensors and Ctuators B,* vol. 257, pp. 228-236, 2018.
[http://dx.doi.org/10.1016/j.snb.2017.10.169]

[59]   Z. Zhang, and S. Ren, "Metal-cluster-based colloidal excimer superstructures", *Angew. Chem. Int. Ed. Engl.,* vol. 55, no. 51, pp. 15708-15710, 2016.
[http://dx.doi.org/10.1002/anie.201608845] [PMID: 27763729]

[60]   R.A. Sperling, and W.J. Parak, "Surface modification, functionalization and bioconjugation of colloidal inorganic nanoparticles", *Philos. Trans.- Royal Soc., Math. Phys. Eng. Sci.,* vol. 368, no. 1915, pp. 1333-1383, 2010.
[http://dx.doi.org/10.1098/rsta.2009.0273] [PMID: 20156828]

[61]   W. Zhow, Y. Y. Zhang, J. Chen, D. Li, J. Zhou, Z. Liu, M. F. Chisholm, S. T. Pantelides, and K. Ping Loh, "Dislocation driven growth of two dimensional lateral quantum well superlattices", *Sci. Adv.,* vol. 4, pp. 1-7, 2018.
[http://dx.doi.org/10.1126/sciadv.aap9096] [PMID: aap9096]

[62]   J. Chen, A. Zheng, Y. Gao, C. He, G. Wu, Y. Chen, X. Kai, and C. Zhu, "Functionalized CdS quantum dots-based luminescence probe for detection of heavy and transition metal ions in aqueous solution", *Spectrochim. Acta A Mol. Biomol. Spectrosc.,* vol. 69, no. 3, pp. 1044-1052, 2008.
[http://dx.doi.org/10.1016/j.saa.2007.06.021] [PMID: 17660001]

[63]   D. Bera, L. Qian, T.-K. Tseng, and P.H. Holloway, *Quantum Dots and Their Multimodal Applications: A Review, Materials,* vol. 3, pp. 2260-2345, 2010.

[64]   J. Kimling, M. Maier, B. Okenve, V. Kotaidis, H. Ballot, and A. Plech, "Turkevich method for gold nanoparticle synthesis revisited", *J. Phys. Chem. B,* vol. 110, no. 32, pp. 15700-15707, 2006.
[http://dx.doi.org/10.1021/jp061667w] [PMID: 16898714]

[65]   M. Reindl, D. Huber, C. Schimpf, S. F. Covre da Silva, and M. B. Rota, "All photonic quantum teleportation using on demnd solid state quantum emitters", *Sci. Adv,* vol. 4, pp. 1-7, 2018.
[PMID: eaau1255]

[66]   J. L. Tambasco, G. Corrielli, R. J. Chapman, A. Crespi, O. Zilberberg, R. Osellame, and A. Peruzzo, "Quantum interference of topological states of light", *Sci. Adv,* pp. 1-5, 2018.
[PMID: eaat3187]

[67] W.W. Chow, and S. Reitzenstein, "Quantum-optical influences in optoelectronics— An introduction", *Appl. Phys. Rev.,* vol. 5, no. 041302, pp. 1-22, 2018.

[68] K.-Hong Luo, S. Brauner, C. Eigner, P. R. Sharapova, and R. Ricken, "Nonlinear integrated quantum electro-optic circuits", *Sci. Adv,* vol. 5, pp. 1-7, 2019.
[http://dx.doi.org/] [PMID: eaat1451]

[69] J. Fenga, Y. Taoa, X. Shena, H. Jinc, T. Zhoub, Y. Zhoub, L. Hua, L. Dan, M. Surong, and L. Yong-Ill, "Highly sensitive and selective fluorescent sensor for tetrabromobisphenol-A in electronic waste samples using molecularly imprinted polymer coated quantum dots", *Microchem. J.,* vol. 144, pp. 93-101, 2019.
[http://dx.doi.org/10.1016/j.microc.2018.08.041]

[70] M.X. Zhao, Q. Xia, X.D. Feng, X.H. Zhu, Z.W. Mao, L.N. Ji, and K. Wang, "Synthesis, biocompatibility and cell labeling of L-arginine-functional beta-cyclodextrin-modified quantum dot probes", *Biomaterials,* vol. 31, no. 15, pp. 4401-4408, 2010.
[http://dx.doi.org/10.1016/j.biomaterials.2010.01.114] [PMID: 20189641]

[71] "Quantum dots: synthesis, bioapplications, and toxicity", *Nanoscale Res Lett,* vol. 480, pp. 1-14, 2012.

[72] W.L. Barnes, A. Dereux, and T.W. Ebbesen, "Surface plasmon subwavelength optics", *Nature,* vol. 424, no. 6950, pp. 824-830, 2003.
[http://dx.doi.org/10.1038/nature01937] [PMID: 12917696]

[73] Y-J. Lu, C-Y. Wang, J. Kim, H-Y. Chen, M-Y. Lu, Y-C. Chen, W-H. Chang, L-J. Chen, M.I. Stockman, C-K. Shih, and S. Gwo, "All-color plasmonic nanolasers with ultralow thresholds: autotuning mechanism for single-mode lasing", *Nano Lett.,* vol. 14, no. 8, pp. 4381-4388, 2014.
[http://dx.doi.org/10.1021/nl501273u] [PMID: 25029207]

[74] L. Ye, Y. Xiao, Y. Liu, and L. Zhang, "G. Cai1, Q. Huo Liu, Strongly Confined Spoof Surface Plasmon Polaritons Waveguiding Enabled by Planar Staggered Plasmonic Waveguides, Scientific Reports", *Nature,* vol. 6, no. 38528, pp. 1-8, 2016.

[75] M. Paulsen, S. Jahns, and M. Gerken, "Intensity based readout of resonant waveguide grating biosensors: systems and nanostructures", *Photonics and Nanostructures-Fundamental and Applications,* vol. 26, pp. 69-79, 2017.
[http://dx.doi.org/10.1016/j.photonics.2017.07.003]

[76] E.C. Kinzel, and X. Xu, "High efficiency excitation of plasmonic waveguides with vertically integrated resonant bowtie apertures", *Opt. Express,* vol. 17, no. 10, pp. 8036-8045, 2009.
[http://dx.doi.org/10.1364/OE.17.008036] [PMID: 19434135]

[77] H. Wei, and H. Xu, "Plasmonic in composite nanostructures", *Mater. Today,* vol. 17, no. 8, pp. 372-380, 2014.
[http://dx.doi.org/10.1016/j.mattod.2014.05.012]

CHAPTER 3

Design, Synthesis and Tuning of Advanced Nanomaterial

Abstract: The design and development of advanced nanomaterials were revised on the basis of the synthesis of organic and inorganic materials for the fabrication of different nanocomposites and hybrid nanomaterials so as to develop advanced applications by the right tuning of each material constituent. It also was discussed how, from the combination of individual materials, metamaterials with new final macroscopic properties could be designed.

Keywords: Advanced nanomaterial, Hybrid nanoarchitecture, Inorganic material, Metamaterial, Organic nanocomposite, Polymeric nanomaterial.

1. CONCEPT OF TUNING OF NANOMATERIAL

In order to develop advanced nanomaterials, we should consider the main properties of the different existing materials based on variable physical and chemical properties used as strategies for targeted applications, as well as the main role of inter-disciplinary research work for nanotechnological developments [1]. Then, by determining special needs, challenges and improvements that should be overcome for the different fields [2, 3], the tuning of matters provided new synthetic alternatives based on the intrinsic properties of the material studied. Thus, the matter composition obtained by combining different existing compatible elements led to varied types of materials.

Accordingly, optical, laser, plasmonic, quantic, conductive, semi-conductive, super-conductive, support, luminescent, biocompatible, biodegradable, printable and wearable materials, among others, were developed and opened up new perspectives in advanced sciences [4]. In addition, advances in biotechnology with the incorporation of biostructures within bioprocesses, the synthesis and development of engineered nanobiostructures and genetically modified biostructures [5] are currently in progress. The combination of the different types of materials also led to new metamaterials properties [6] Finally, the production of new tools such as lasers combining the right tuning of materials for instrumentation and light was awarded the last Nobel Prize in Physics 2018 shared by France, Canada and USA [7].

2. ORGANIC NANOCOMPOSITE

Organic nanocomposites based on different organic materials and organic chemical reactions have allowed the design, synthesis and development of varied and versatile material properties based on their intrinsic characteristics, in addition to the final properties achieved from their interaction. These materials could be obtained from a large number of organic chemical reactions in different media, generating defined nanoarchitectures in colloidal dispersions, nanoaggregates, modified surfaces and fibers and porous, biodegradable and crosslinked material. Therefore, these nanocomposites and materials could function as devices where other types of materials and properties could be incorporated as well.

The electronic characteristics of the organic molecules define the type of reactions that could be applied, as well as their functionality and interaction with their environment. In this way, fluorescent properties, electron transfer reactions and conductive, thermo-sensitive properties, among others, could be developed for targeted applications.

Accordingly, organic nanomaterials have been reported and applied in different fields, as in self-assembled fluorescent molecules for bioimaging generation [8]. These nanoassemblies were based on non-covalent interaction between molecular assemblers such as short polymeric chains that incorporated different highly conjugated organic molecules in order to obtain highly fluorescent organics dots. These nanoassemblies were also produced exo-*in situ* of applications as well as in-situ based on hydrophobic effect, polarities, pH modifications, *etc*. Even if the polymers were highly applied to the development of the nanostructure, the use of short molecular spacers and multi-functional molecular linkers should also be stressed.

Moreover, based on the condensation of dextrans at high temperatures, carbon nanodots showed to be a versatile cargo of different types of inorganic [9] and organic [10] fluorophores. These types of organic nanomaterials were considered as new photoluminescent labellers with reduced size, comparable (1–4 nm) to quantum dots. In addition, from cyanobacteria, bio-carbonaceous dots showed cargo properties of doxorubicin for drug delivery and imaging application in cancer cells [11].

Another type of nanoarchitecture, based on high conjugated organic molecules such as molecular cores grafted with short molecular shells by covalent linking of poly-ethylene glycol and poly-esters, synthesized fluorescent organic core-shell nanoparticles and applied to cell staining applications [12]. This nanoarchitecture approach of the molecular core could be extended to a large molecular library of new fluorescent multifunctional molecules, such as the recently reported bioinspired synthesis of polyfunctional indoles [13]. In order to mention the importance of organic molecules, not only as molecular templates, but also as bio-interactions, we could mention the dextran-coated superparamagnetic iron oxide nanoparticles, with 20 times higher entry within pancreatic cells and drug delivery [14] than that with no sugar coating. Similarly, we could mention the multi-functional molecular structures by new reaction pathways involving bond activations such as valuable C-O bond for linking and cleavage of organic fibers such as mimetic of lignin [15]. These types of material architecture could be applied as a material of support for the preparation of fiber-like nanomaterial, for example, mimic multilayered structure of organic electronic devices on individual polymer chains [16], where electronic holes and shuttlers should be generated through different strategies and approaches.

We should also recognize the importance of the uses of non-covalent interactions of supramolecular systems [17] and DNA [18] for supramolecular nanoparticles [19] and origamis nanoarchitectures [20, 21], respectively.

Hence, the wide diversity of organic molecules and their chemistry showed to be particularly useful for the design and synthesis of new multifunctional organic material with a high impact on applied organic nanocomposites and materials in diverse fields.

3. POLYMERIC NANOMATERIAL

Like organic nanocomposites, organic polymeric and inorganic materials based on organic and inorganic chemical reactions produced stable nanomaterials, biodegradable nanoparticles in colloidal dispersions, films and many properties that have allowed a large number of advanced nanomaterials and applications in different fields. As a result, several approaches have been developed on the basis of organic film polymerization for targeted functionalization by appropriate tuning of the different components.

Depending on their intrinsic material composition, varied macroscopic properties were exploited, including flexible polymers for multifunctional applications and wearable devices such as flexible sensors [22]. Organic polymers such as (PEN) [23], polyimide (PI) [24], parylene [25] and polypirrole [26] showed excellent flexible properties, allowing the adaptation over different surface topographies. In addition, transparent, flexible and thin sensor surfaces for passive light-point localization based on two functional polymers [27] can be reported, using poly(vinylidene fluoride) (PVDF) and poly(3,4-ethylene dioxythiophene): polystyrenesulfonic acid (PEDOT:PSS) as active transparent materials for sensor design.

As regards inorganic polymers, the process and material properties of polydimethylsiloxane (PDMS) for optical micro-electro-mechanical systems (MEMS) [28] generated high technological applications, such as wearable wireless electrochemical signaling with bio-potential acquisition [29] and compliant and stretchable thermoelectric coils for energy harvesting in miniature flexible devices [30].

Applications also include emerging flexible and wearable physical sensing platforms for healthcare and biomedicine [31] as well as wearable organic optoelectronic sensors for medicine [32]; conductive polymers for printed electronics [33]; and stretchable organic optoelectronics [34] and epidermal microfluidic devices for sweat collection, biomarker and thermogravimetric analysis in an aquatic setting [35].

In addition to variable polymeric surface thickness, depending on monomer composition and reaction media, varied sizes and shapes of nanoparticles in colloidal media [36] have been obtained. According to monomeric composition and final properties generated, several physical and chemical properties enabled the detection and tracking of these nanoparticles, as in the case of polystyrene beads that showed well-defined nanostructures with particular electronic properties allowing manipulation by electrophoresis [37]. Moreover, by varying copolymer composition, it was possible to modify and tune their properties and nanoarchitecture. For instance, from a polymeric core template [38], defined multi-structured nanoparticles were obtained by Atom Transfer Radical Polymerization (ATRP), capable of generating different nanostructures by the self-assembly properties of the segmented copolymers [39] used. Similarly, copolymers of poly(butyl acrylate) with polyacrylonitrile led to spherical, cylindrical or lamellar morphologies, depending on the block copolymer composition.

Additionally, the design and synthesis of new nanostructures based on short biopeptides and biomolecules gave way to the templated synthesis of small bio-nanoparticles with potential future applications in *vivo* due to their low toxicity. In these types of grafted or modified cores, IgM pentamers and hexamers showed asymmetric and symmetric particles [40] for potential templated designs.

Moreover, the application of hydrolysable esters from different organic acids that act as functional monomers and generated biodegradable nanoparticles *via* esterification reactions should also be considered. This type of nanomaterials includes poly-galic acid (PLGA) [41], malic acid [42], lactic acid (PL) [43] and copolymers [44] that proved to be versatile nanoplatforms for cargo, bioimaging and drug delivery applications [45].

Finally, we should also include hydrogel material potentially applied to regenerative medicine and drug delivery, and be incorporated in micro- and nanodevices. Cases in point include gelatin-based hydrogel sensors through homobifunctional triazolinediones targeting tyrosine residues [46] and smart pH-responsive fluorescent hydrogels using a new thioflavin T crosslinker [47]. Even if hydrogels showed low toxicity depending on their composition, this issue still poses a challenge by developments of hydrogel based on biogenic molecules [48]. In a similar way, supramolecular interactions enabled the non-covalent linking of different parts of supramolecular nanoparticles [49, 50], as well as the formation of hierarchical self-assemblies, such as N-annulated perylenes that generated nano-patterned surfaces [51], with many potential uses in functionalized surfaces within micro- and nanodevice fabrications.

4. INORGANIC NANOMATERIAL

There is a huge number of inorganic nanomaterials classified according to their physical, chemical properties and applications in different types of materials. These materials showed high versatility on the nanoscale control as well as incorporation in surfaces, arrays, films and alloys for advanced nanomaterial developments. Such nanomaterials added different properties in view of the intrinsic material composition; thus, particular properties were generated from the nanoscale. These inorganic materials could be obtained by different methodologies in colloidal dispersion with wet-chemical procedures and by nanolithography techniques as well.

Within the UV region, and on the basis of their electronic properties, aluminium nanoparticles [52] are used as substrates for Metal Enhanced Fluorescence (**MEF**) in the ultraviolet for the label-free detection of biomolecules [53] and In^0 nanoparticles with tuned particle size and high oxidation stability [54] with potential application in nanoimaging.

For longer wavelengths depending on size and shape, gold nanoparticles showed/proved to be useful for colorimetric and fluorescent detection of ions and small organic molecules [55] and biocompatible applications such as drug delivery, nanoimaging and bioimaging [56]. In addition, silver [57] nanoparticles showed stronger plasmonic properties having numerous uses, including biosensors [58], nanoimaging [59] and antifungal nanomaterials [60]. Copper nanoparticles showed different applications from conductive to superconductivity properties [61], sensor nanoplatforms [62] and antibacterial agents [63].

Magnetic nanoparticle synthesis such as Fe_2O_3 nanoparticles in colloidal media [64] allowed developing proofs of concepts related from the control and separation of nanoparticles for different nanoparticles to nanoalloys of Fe doped magnetic nanodiamonds applied such as for MRI agents [65]. These copper and palladium nanoparticles offered effective catalyst materials due to their high surface area to volume ratio and high surface energy [66]. In the same vein, zinc oxide nanoparticles [67] showed potential nanotechnological applications, based on their control of size and shape, luminescent nanomaterials [68], photocatalytic nanoplatforms [69] and new plasmonic multilayered resonators [70].

With these resonant materials, the possibility of synthesis of hollowed nanoparticles in a controlled organized media of colloidal dispersion should be explored, such as gold nanocage structures in biomedicine [71].

Thus, based on the inorganic materials referred to above, different nanoarchitectures and properties could be obtained, as in the synthesis of nanoshells [72] over different nanotemplates, bimetallic gold-silver core-shell nanoparticles [73] with dual properties on single nanoplatforms [74] for nanomedicine applications, nickel–silver core–shell nanoparticles for conductive materials [75] and InGaN/GaN core-shell nanostructures for luminescent semiconductor nanomaterials [76], gold-silver bimetallic nanocluster with precise atomic structure [77] and enhanced luminescent properties in the NIR wavelength interval. In addition, these inorganic nanomaterials could be incorporated into new tandem organic light-emitting diodes [78] and over silica substrates [79] such as optical fibers [80] in the field of nanomedicine [81].

5. HYBRID NANOARCHITECTURE

In order to obtain the targeted functionalization of nanomaterials for advanced applications, hybrid nanoarchitectures could be designed by combining different organic and inorganic components [82]. Accordingly, different properties could be coupled from each part of the nanostructures. Many proofs of concepts of nanomaterials used as nanotools within micro- and Nanodevices and for enhanced performance in advanced instrumentation were reported. In this field, a vast number of developments could be reported; however, we mentioned, in this section, few representative examples of nanomaterials from individual nanoparticles in colloidal dispersion for varied application, modified materials and surfaces with properties related to the transmission of signals for applied wearable material.

Hybrid nanoparticles for chemical sensing based on modified inorganic nanoparticle templates with polymers [83] and short molecular spacers [84] allowed molecular detection and controlled switch on/off drug delivery applications and luminescent properties. Moreover, modified polymeric crosslinked materials with incorporation of supramolecular systems led to drug delivery systems with regulation by mechanical stimuli [85, 86].

Moreover, luminescent quantum dots with several modifications were reported for different uses. For example, modified quantum dots with anti-bodies and biomolecules for biosensing and biolabelling [87], incorporated into lab-on-chips for luminescence routing [88] and combined with carbon nanotubes for thin-film transistors [89].

Besides, the incorporation of different inorganic nanoparticles in different polymeric films produced varied properties in view of the intrinsic characteristics of individual components and interactions, for instance, transparent electrode applied to epidermal electronics based on flexible polydimethylsiloxane (PDMS) and conductive silver nanowire (AgNW) networks [90]. Another case in point comprises high-gain organic electrochemical transistors processed in micro-grid substrates and coating of modified poly(3-methoxypropyl acrylate) (PM3CA) with parylene, gold and poly(3,4-ethylenedioxythiophene) polystyrene sulfonate (PEDOT:PSS) thin layers. Therefore, PM3CA showed blood compatibility and non-thrombogenic properties [91] tested in *vivo* of rat core. On the other hand, fully rubbery integrated electronics allowed highly effective mobility of intrinsically stretchable semiconductors [92] and application of low temperature on conductive copper films on flexible polymer substrates produced sintering of composite Cu Ink in Air [93], potentially applied to enhanced conduction properties. The use of polymers as support should be particularly taken into account to incorporate sensing approaches in textile electronics [94] and wearable health monitoring patches [95].

The production of high-impact material should also include functionalized nanoarchitectures based on nucleic acids and varying DNA strand lengths for targeted/specific applications. Hence, we could mention the molecular engineering of functional nucleic acid nanomaterials in applications in *vivo* [96], folding of DNA to create nanoscale shapes and patterns [97], DNA from natural sources in the design of functional devices [98], bioorganic optoelectronic devices using DNA [99] and DNA origamis [100].

Finally, within functionalized hybrid nanomaterials and nano-patterned surfaces adopting new molecular approaches, in conjunction with the know-how of nanolithography techniques, the case of nanomesh scaffold for supramolecular nanowire optoelectronic devices [101] and metal-organic framework (MOFs) as a protective coating for biodiagnostic chips [102] were reported. In particular, MOFs demonstrated to be versatile porous nanomaterials [103] by precisely controlled formation of ordered vacancies that generated confined platforms for chemical modification, including ligands, linkers, metal exchangers and metalation reactions [104].

6. METAMATERIAL

Metamaterials are synthetic composites with tunable properties such as acoustic, electrical, magnetic, optical and luminescent properties based on the interaction of variable material composition. Nature publishing defined them as engineered structures designed to interact with electromagnetic radiation in the desired fashion. They usually comprise an array of structures smaller than the wavelength of interest. These so-called meta-atoms can interact with the electric and magnetic components of light in a way that natural atoms cannot. Thus, their properties arise from the interaction of different atoms that produce new properties in comparison to individual atoms whose components are derived from original materials [105]. These types of nanomaterials are not just hybrid nanoarchitectures; they are synthetic and tunable materials where different properties are kept in contact within the near field and new ones in the farfield. For such reasons, many studies center on these types of new nanomaterials at different levels, from atomic to nano- and microscales, such as research into few photon-matter interactions to electron-optics, where the quantic phenomena should be considered in order to explain the behaviour of electron within confined porous metamaterials [106].

Similarly, the electromagnetic fields generated in the near field of nanostructured surfaces, films and nanocomposites could produce different interactions with their environment, in addition to a generation of new properties of the materials, as in the design of nano-imprinted colloids such as nanoantennas for ultrathin light polarizing plasmonic metasurfaces [107]. This type of metallic arrays could be applied to the generation of non-classical light based on modified metasurfaces with targeted excitations. For example, from studies related to dielectric nanorod scattering and its influence on material interfaces [108], it was observed that from the high scattering produced by these types of nanoarchitectures, the control of light propagation could be exerted across material interfaces. Thus ZnO nanorods showed excellent antenna-like resonance, which can be used to control light coupling and propagation. These metasurfaces can be tuned at different wavelengths for applications based on the right combination of nanostructured surfaces and light excitation, coupled to molecular switchers that allow surface control. For example, a molecular switcher in the near-45 infrared interval to activate the responsive dynamic of wrinkle patterns [109] from modified surfaces.

Based on light interaction between metamaterials and light, molecular chirality sensing and new imaging modes were developed, such as circular dichroism (CD) [110] spectroscopy, consisting of measuring the difference in the absorption of two opposite circularly polarized light modes, and optical chirality enhancement [111] based on the interaction of molecules within modified metasurfaces. For fluorescent molecules, fluorescence detected circular dichroism [112] (FDCD) was also developed, potentially applied also to the modified metasurfaces described above. The CD and FDCD were used extensively to study conformational changes in macromolecules. The CD technique measures the difference in absorption for left and right circularly polarized light. The FDCD technique detects the same difference by measuring the variation of the fluorescence intensity excited by left and right circularly polarized light [113]. Moreover, spectrally selective chiral silicon metasurfaces based on infrared fano-resonance [114] can also be mentioned, where the high sensitivity of fano-resonance was demonstrated with molecular asymmetries for molecular sensing.

In relation to imaging and microscopy, metamaterial superlenses operating at a visible wavelength for imaging applications [115] should also be discussed. These superlens consist of gallium phosphide (GaP) dielectric slab waveguides with a hexagonal array of silver rods embedded within the GaP dielectric material.

Moreover, from light interaction with varied metasurface conformation, dynamic holography and optical information encryption were generated [116] (Fig. **1**).

These tuneable metamaterials have potential applications in advanced microscopy techniques such as photon-induced near-field electron microscopy (PINEM)[117], according to the capturing of the evanescent field on its intrinsic time scale (femtoseconds); and where the nanomaterial constitution has the main role on image generation.

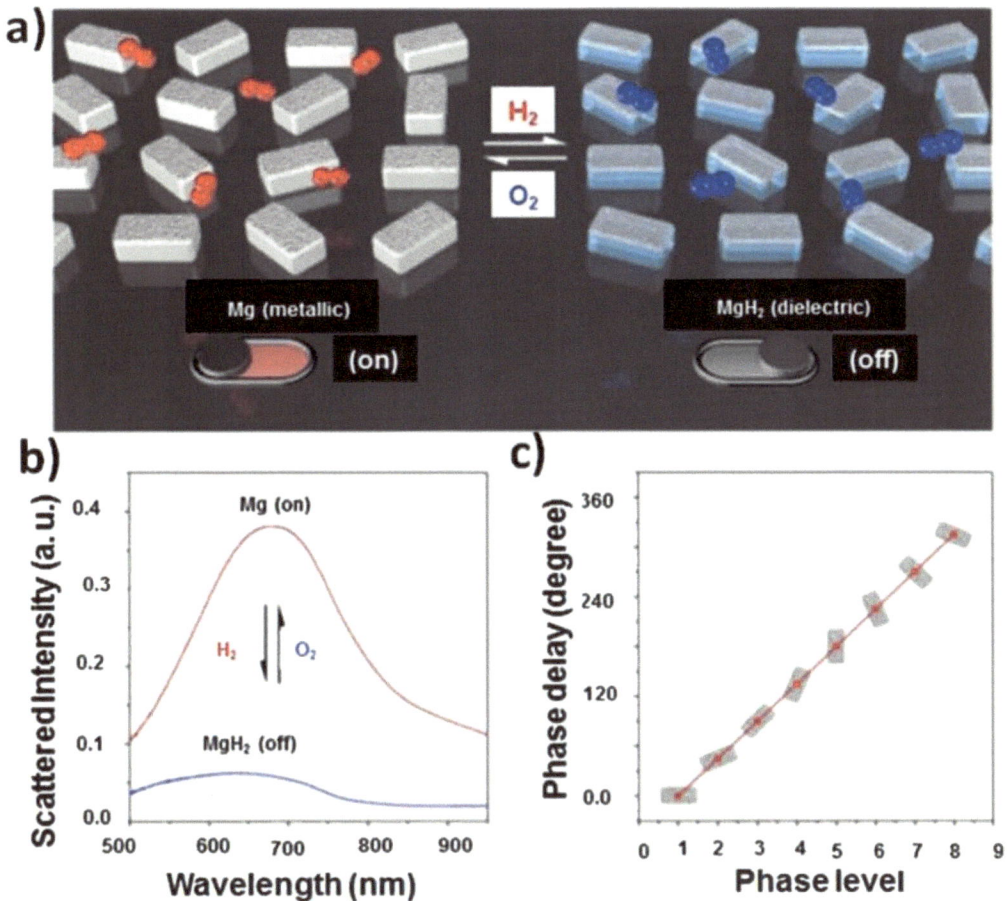

Fig. (1). Working principle of the dynamic metasurface pixels. **a)** Schema of hydrogen-responsive Mg nanorods (200 nm × 80 nm × 50 nm), sandwiched between a Ti (5 nm)/Pd (10 nm) capping layer and a Ti (3 nm) adhesion layer. **b)** Measured scattering spectra of such nanorod in Mg (on) and MgH (off) states. Before hydrogenation, the Mg nanorod exhibits a strong plasmonic resonance (red curve); after hydrogenation (10% H), the MgH rod shows a nearly feature less spectrum (blue curve). The process is reversible through dehydrogenation using O (20%). a.u., arbitrary units. **c)** Simulated phase delay for the different phase levels. The orientation of the nanorod at each phase level is shown [116].

Another property that needs to be discussed is the generation of tuneable thermal capabilities of semiconductor metasurface resonators [118]. For example, by tuning Si and Ge single resonators and metasurfaces, large temperature ranges 80–873 K were caused, with temperature-dependence with resonance frequency. These properties were derived from thin epitaxial grown InAs active and reflector layers by optically pumping with 980 nm pulse laser and voltage excitations [119].

Finally, on the basis of the right tuning of metamaterials, we could report variable mechanical strengths [120], 3D active mechanical mesostructures based on varied wafer composition, gold and polymeric film deposition and etching [121], porous membranes based on carbon nanotubes with sub-1.27 nm pores [122] and tunable shapes, volumes against external response, based on polymeric nanomaterials, that arouse special interest in tissue engineering, biosensing, flexible displays and soft robotics [123].

CONCLUDING REMARKS

Advanced nanomaterials were developed from different properties of organic and inorganic materials that contributed to the final targeted properties. Thus, different nanomaterials were used as templates for the bottom-up and nanoengineering, including inorganic nanoparticles joined to different polymers, organic molecules, supra-structures and biostructures. In addition, with the accurate development of the material property of each component of the whole nanomaterial, new advanced and enhanced metamaterial properties were developed.

REFERENCES

[1] A.L. Porter, and J. Youtie, "Nanotecnology research directions for societal needs in 2020, How interdisciplinary is nanotechnology?", *Nanopart Res,* vol. 11, pp. 1023-1041, 2009.
[http://dx.doi.org/10.1007/s11051-009-9607-0]

[2] K. Ariga, K. Minami, M. Ebara, and J. Nakanishi, "What are the emerging concepts and challenges in NANO, Nanoarchitectonics, hand-operating nanotechnology and mechanobiology", *Polym. J.,* vol. 48, pp. 371-389, 2016.
[http://dx.doi.org/10.1038/pj.2016.8]

[3] M. C. Roco, C. A. Mirkin, and M. C. Hersam, Springer. Dordrecht Heidelberg London New York,

[4] J. Berg, "Editorial: science advances advancing", *Science,* vol. 361, no. 6397, p. 7, 2018.

[5] T. Li, C. Zhang, K.L. Yang, and J. He, "Unique genetic cassettes in a Thermoanaerobacterium contribute to simultaneous conversion of cellulose and mono sugars into butanol", *Sci. Adv.,* vol. 4, no. e1701475, pp. 1-12, 2018.

[6] J. Li, S. Kamin, G. Zheng, F. Neubrech, S. Zhang, and N. Liu, *Sci. Adv,* vol. 4, no. eaar6768 15, pp. 1-7, 2018.

[7] A. Ashkin, G. Mourou, and D. Strickland, "The Nobel Prize in Physics 2018, for Tools made of light: groundbreaking inventions in the field of laser physics", *Press Release from The Royal Swedish Academy of Science,* 2018.

[8] K. Zhang, Y-J. Gao, P-P. Yang, G-B. Qi, J-P. Zhang, L. Wang, and H. Wang, "Self-Assembled Fluorescent Organic Nanomaterials for Biomedical Imaging", *Adv. Healthc. Mater.,* vol. 7, no. 20, p. e1800344, 2018.
[http://dx.doi.org/10.1002/adhm.201800344] [PMID: 30137689]

[9] A.M. Vostrikova, A.A. Kokorina, P.A. Demina, and S.V. German, "Fabrication and photoluminescent properties of Tb3+ doped carbon nanodots, Scientific Reports", *Nature,* vol. 8, no. 16301, pp. 1-8, 2018.

[10] L. Shi, J.H. Yang, H.B. Zeng, Y.M. Chen, S.C. Yang, C. Wu, H. Zeng, O. Yoshihito, and Q. Zhang, "Carbon dots with high fluorescence quantum yield: the fluorescence originates from organic

fluorophores", *Nanoscale,* vol. 8, no. 30, pp. 14374-14378, 2016.
[http://dx.doi.org/10.1039/C6NR00451B] [PMID: 27426926]

[11]   H. Uk Lee, S.Y. Park, E. Sik Park, B. Son, S. Chang Lee, J. Won Lee, Y-C. Lee, K. Suk Kang, M.I. Kim, H. Gyu Park, S. Choi, and Y. Suk Huh, "Photoluminescent carbon nanotags from harmful cyanobacteria for drug delivery and imaging in cancer cells", *Sci. Rep.,* vol. 4, no. 4665, pp. 1-7, 2014.

[12]   M. Yin, J. Shen, R. Gropeanu, G.O. Pflugfelder, T. Weil, and K. Müllen, "Fluorescent core/shell nanoparticles for specific cell-nucleus staining", *Small,* vol. 4, no. 7, pp. 894-898, 2008.
[http://dx.doi.org/10.1002/smll.200701107] [PMID: 18561214]

[13]   Z. Huang, O. Kwon, H. Huang, A. Fadli, X. Marat, M. Moreau, and J-P. Lumb, "A bioinspired synthesis of polyfunctional indoles", *Angew. Chem. Int. Ed. Engl.,* vol. 57, no. 37, pp. 11963-11967, 2018.
[http://dx.doi.org/10.1002/anie.201806490] [PMID: 29978600]

[14]   M.P. Arachchige, S.S. Laha, A.R. Naik, K.T. Lewis, R. Naik, and B.P. Jena, "Functionalized nanoparticles enable tracking the rapid entry and release of doxorubicin in human pancreatic cancer cells", *Micron,* vol. 92, pp. 25-31, 2017.
[http://dx.doi.org/10.1016/j.micron.2016.10.005] [PMID: 27846432]

[15]   Q. Mei, Y. Yang, H. Liu, S. Li, H. Liu, and B. Han, "A new route to synthesize aryl acetates from carbonylation of aryl methyl ethers", *Sci. Adv,* vol. 4, no. eaaq0266, pp. 1-7, 2018.

[16]   C.M. Tonge, E.R. Sauvé, S. Cheng, T.A. Howard, and Z.M. Hudson, "Multiblock bottlebrush nanofibers from organic electronic materials", *J. Am. Chem. Soc.,* vol. 140, no. 37, pp. 11599-11603, 2018.
[http://dx.doi.org/10.1021/jacs.8b07915] [PMID: 30180557]

[17]   J-M. Lehn, "From supramolecular chemistry towards constitutional dynamic chemistry and adaptive chemistry", *Chem. Soc. Rev.,* vol. 36, no. 2, pp. 151-160, 2007.
[http://dx.doi.org/10.1039/B616752G] [PMID: 17264919]

[18]   Y.C. Hung, D.M. Bauer, I. Ahmed, and L. Fruk, "DNA from natural sources in design of functional devices", *Methods,* vol. 67, no. 2, pp. 105-115, 2014.
[http://dx.doi.org/10.1016/j.ymeth.2014.03.003] [PMID: 24631889]

[19]   J. W. Steed, and P. A. Gale, "Nanotechnology, supramolecular nanoparticles", *Supramolecular Chemistry: From Molecules to Nanomaterials,* vol. 8, pp. 1-4014, 2012.

[20]   K. Doré, R. Neagu-Plesu, M. Leclerc, D. Boudreau, and A.M. Ritcey, "Characterization of superlighting polymer-DNA aggregates: a fluorescence and light scattering study", *Langmuir,* vol. 23, no. 1, pp. 258-264, 2007.
[http://dx.doi.org/10.1021/la061699a] [PMID: 17190512]

[21]   G. Tikhomirov, P. Petersen, and L. Qian, "Fractal assembly of micrometre-scale DNA origami arrays with arbitrary patterns", *Nature,* vol. 552, no. 7683, pp. 67-71, 2017.
[http://dx.doi.org/10.1038/nature24655] [PMID: 29219965]

[22]   A. Nag, MMukhopadhyay S. C., and J. Kosel, "Wereable flexible sensors: A Review", *IEEE Sens. J,* vol. 17, no. 13, pp. 3949-3960, 2017.
[http://dx.doi.org/10.1109/JSEN.2017.2705700]

[23]   T. Someya, and T. Sekitani, "Bionic skins using flexible organic devices", *Proc. ESSDERC,* 2014pp. 68-71

[24]   Y. Qin, Q. Peng, Y. Ding, Z. Lin, C. Wang, Y. Li, F. Xu, J. Li, Y. Yuan, X. He, and Y. Li, "Lightweight, superelastic, and mechanically flexible graphene/polyimide nanocomposite foam for strain sensor application", *ACS Nano,* vol. 9, no. 9, pp. 8933-8941, 2015.
[http://dx.doi.org/10.1021/acsnano.5b02781] [PMID: 26301319]

[25]   D. Ha, W.N. de Vries, S.W.M. John, P.P. Irazoqui, and W.J. Chappell, "Polymer-based miniature flexible capacitive pressure sensor for intraocular pressure (IOP) monitoring inside a mouse eye",

Biomed. Microdevices, vol. 14, no. 1, pp. 207-215, 2012.
[http://dx.doi.org/10.1007/s10544-011-9598-3] [PMID: 21987004]

[26]   A.P. Tjahyono, "A five-fingered hand exoskeleton driven by pneumatic article-title muscles with novel polypyrrole sensors, Ind. Robot", *Int. J.,* vol. 40, no. 3, pp. 51-260, 2013.

[27]   G. Buchberger, R.A. Barb, J. Schoeftner, S. Bauer, W. Hilberg, B. Mayrhofer, and B. Jakoby, "Transparent, flexible, thin sensor surfaces for passive light point localization based on two functional polymers", *Sens. Actuators A Phys.,* vol. 239, pp. 70-78, 2016.
[http://dx.doi.org/10.1016/j.sna.2016.01.007]

[28]   F. Schneider, J. Draheim, R. Kamberger, and U. Wallrabe, "Process and material properties of polydimethylsiloxane (PDMS) for Optical MEMS", *Sens. Actuators A Phys.,* vol. 151, pp. 95-99, 2009.
[http://dx.doi.org/10.1016/j.sna.2009.01.026]

[29]   C-Y. Chen, C-L. Chang, T-F. Chien, and C-H. Luo, "Flexible PDMS electrode for one-point wearable wireless bio-potential acquisition", *Sens. Actuators A Phys.,* vol. 203, pp. 20-28, 2013.
[http://dx.doi.org/10.1016/j.sna.2013.08.010]

[30]   K. Nan, S. D. Kang, K. Li, K. J. Yu, F. Zhu, J. Wang, A. C. Dunn, C. Zhou, Z. Xie, M. T. Agne, H. Wang, H. Luan, Y. Zhang, Y. Huang, G. J. Snyder, and J. A. Rogers, "Compliant and stretchable thermoelectric coils for energy harvesting in miniature flexible devices", *Sci. Adv,* vol. 4, no. eaau5849, pp. 1-7, 2018.

[31]   J.C.Yeo Kenry, and C. Teck Lim, "Emerging flexible and wearable physical sensing platforms for healthcare and biomedical applications, Microsystems & Nanoengineering", *Nature,* vol. 2, no. 16043, pp. 1-19, 2016.

[32]   A.K. Bansal, S. Hou, O. Kulyk, E.M. Bowman, and I.D.W. Samuel, "Wearable Organic Optoelectronic Sensors for Medicine", *Adv. Mater.,* vol. 27, no. 46, pp. 7638-7644, 2015.
[http://dx.doi.org/10.1002/adma.201403560] [PMID: 25488890]

[33]   A. Kamyshny, and S. Magdassi, "Conductive nanomaterials for printed electronics", *Small,* vol. 10, no. 17, pp. 3515-3535, 2014.
[http://dx.doi.org/10.1002/smll.201303000] [PMID: 25340186]

[34]   Y. Lee, J. Y. Oh, W. Xu, O. Kim, T. Roy Kim, J. Kang, Y. Kim, D. Son, J. B. H. Tok, M. J. Park, Z. Bao, and T. W. Lee, "Stretchable organic optoelectronic sensorimotor synapse", *Sci Adv,* vol. 4, no. eaat7387, pp. 1-9, 2018.

[35]   J. T. Reeder, J. Choi, Y. Hue, P. Gutruf, J. Hanson, M. Liu, T. Ray, A. J. Bandodkar, R. Avila, W. Xia, S. Krishman, S. Xu, K. Barnes, M. Pahnke, R. Ghaffari, Y. Huang, and J. J. A. Rogers, "Waterproof, electronics-enabled, epidermal microfluidic devices for sweat collection, biomarker analysis, and thermogravimetric in aquatic setting", *Sci Adv,* vol. 5, no. eaau6356, pp. 1-13, 2019.

[36]   J. Prasad Rao, and K. E. Geckeler, "Polymer nanoparticles: preparation techniques and size control parameters", *Progress in Polymer Science,* vol. 36, no. 7, pp. 887-913, 2011.

[37]   Q. Chen, and Y.J. Yuan, "A Review of Polystirene bead manipulation by dielectrophoresis", *RSC Advances,* vol. 9, pp. 4963-4981, 2019.
[http://dx.doi.org/10.1039/C8RA09017C]

[38]   M. Szczęch, and K. Szczepanowicz, "Polymeric core-shell nanoparticles prepared by spontaneous emulsification solvent evaporation and functionalized by the layer-by-layer method", *Nanomaterials (Basel),* vol. 10, no. 3, pp. 1-16, 2020.
[http://dx.doi.org/10.3390/nano10030496] [PMID: 32164194]

[39]   T. Kowalewski, R.D. McCullough, and K. Matyjaszewski, "Complex nanostructured copolymers prepared by ATRP", *European Physical Journal,* vol. 10, no. 1, pp. 5-16, 2003.
[PMID: 15011074]

[40]   E. Hiramoto, A. Tsutsumi, R. Suzuki, S. Matsuoka, and S. Arai, "The IgM pentamer is an asymmetric

pentagon with an open groove that binds the AIM protein", *Sci. Adv,* vol. 4, no. eaau1199, pp. 1-9, 2018.

[41] H. Xie, and J.W. Smith, "Fabrication of PLGA nanoparticles with a fluidic nanoprecipitation system", *J. Nanobiotechnology,* vol. 8, no. 18, p. 18, 2010.
[http://dx.doi.org/10.1186/1477-3155-8-18] [PMID: 20707919]

[42] A. Lanz-Landázuri, J. Portilla-Arias, A. Martínez de Ilarduya, M. García-Alvarez, E. Holler, J. Ljubimova, and S. Muñoz-Guerra, "Nanoparticles of esterified polymalic acid for controlled anticancer drug release", *Macromol. Biosci.,* vol. 14, no. 9, pp. 1325-1336, 2014.
[http://dx.doi.org/10.1002/mabi.201400124] [PMID: 24902676]

[43] M.L. Hans, and A.M. Lowman, "Biodegradable nanoparticles for Drug delivery and targeting", *Curr. Opin. Solid State Mater. Sci.,* vol. 6, pp. 319-327, 2002.
[http://dx.doi.org/10.1016/S1359-0286(02)00117-1]

[44] D.P. Go, S.L. Gras, D. Mitra, T.H. Nguyen, G.W. Stevens, J.J. Cooper-White, and A.J. O'Connor, "Multilayered microspheres for the controlled release of growth factors in tissue engineering", *Biomacromolecules,* vol. 12, no. 5, pp. 1494-1503, 2011.
[http://dx.doi.org/10.1021/bm1014574] [PMID: 21413682]

[45] C.P. Reis, R.J. Neufeld, A.J. Ribeiro, and F. Veiga, "Nanoencapsulation I. Methods for preparation of drug-loaded polymeric nanoparticles", *Nanomedicine (Lond.),* vol. 2, no. 1, pp. 8-21, 2006.
[http://dx.doi.org/10.1016/j.nano.2005.12.003] [PMID: 17292111]

[46] R. Guizzardi, L. Vaghi, M. Marelli, A. Natalello, I. Andreosso, A. Papagni, and L. Cipolla, "Gelatin-Based Hydrogels through Homobifunctional Triazolinediones Targeting Tyrosine Residues", *Molecules,* vol. 24, no. 3, pp. 1-12, 2019.
[http://dx.doi.org/10.3390/molecules24030589] [PMID: 30736414]

[47] Z. Xiao, R. Andrew Lennox Wylie, E. Ruth, L. Brisson, and L. Andrew Connal, "pH-responsive fluorescent hydrogels using a new thioflavin t cross-linker", *J. Polym. Sci. A Polym. Chem.,* vol. 54, pp. 591-595, 2016.
[http://dx.doi.org/10.1002/pola.27974]

[48] L. Xu, C. Wang, Y. Cui, A. Li, Y. Li, and D. Qiu, "Conjoined network rendered stiff and though hydrogels from biogenic molecules", *Sci. Adv,* vol. 5, no. eaau344, pp. 1-9, 2019.

[49] M.W. Ambrogio, T.A. Pecorelli, K. Patel, N.M. Khashab, A. Trabolsi, H.A. Khatib, Y.Y. Botros, J.I. Zink, and J.F. Stoddart, "Snap-top nanocarriers", *Org. Lett.,* vol. 12, no. 15, pp. 3304-3307, 2010.
[http://dx.doi.org/10.1021/ol101286a] [PMID: 20608669]

[50] D. Gontero, M. Lessard-Viger, D. Brouard, A.G. Bracamonte, D. Boudreau, and A.V. Veglia, "Smart multifunctional nanoparticles design as sensors and drug delivery systems based on supramolecular chemistry", *Microchem. J.,* vol. 130, pp. 316-328, 2017.
[http://dx.doi.org/10.1016/j.microc.2016.10.007]

[51] E.E. Greciano, B. Matarranz, and L. Sanchez, *Pathway Complexity Versus Hierarchical Self-Assembly in NAnnulated Perylenes:Structural Effects in Seeded Supramolecular Polymerization, Angew.* 57th ed. Chem. Int, 2018, pp. 4697-4701.

[52] M.J. Meziani, C.E. Bunker, F. Lu, H. Li, W. Wang, E.A. Guliants, R.A. Quinn, and Y.P. Sun, "Formation and properties of stabilized aluminum nanoparticles", *ACS Appl. Mater. Interfaces,* vol. 1, no. 3, pp. 703-709, 2009.
[http://dx.doi.org/10.1021/am800209m] [PMID: 20355993]

[53] M.H. Chowdhury, K. Ray, S.K. Gray, J. Pond, and J.R. Lakowicz, "Aluminum nanoparticles as substrates for metal-enhanced fluorescence in the ultraviolet for the label-free detection of biomolecules", *Anal. Chem.,* vol. 81, no. 4, pp. 1397-1403, 2009.
[http://dx.doi.org/10.1021/ac802118s] [PMID: 19159327]

[54] C. Kind, and C. Feldmann, "One-pot synthesis of in0 nanoparticles with tuned particle size and high

oxidation stability", *Chem. Mater.,* vol. 23, pp. 4982-4987, 2011.
[http://dx.doi.org/10.1021/cm202256t]

[55]   D. Liu, Z. Wang, and X. Jiang, "Gold nanoparticles for the colorimetric and fluorescent detection of ions and small organic molecules", *Nanoscale,* vol. 3, no. 4, pp. 1421-1433, 2011.
[http://dx.doi.org/10.1039/c0nr00887g] [PMID: 21359318]

[56]   D.T. Nguyen, D.J. Kim, and K.S. Kim, "Controlled synthesis and biomolecular probe application of gold nanoparticles", *Micron,* vol. 42, no. 3, pp. 207-227, 2011.
[http://dx.doi.org/10.1016/j.micron.2010.09.008] [PMID: 20952201]

[57]   B. Wiley, Y. Sun, B. Mayers, and Y. Xia, "Shape-controlled synthesis of metal nanostructures: the case of silver", *Chemistry,* vol. 11, no. 2, pp. 454-463, 2005.
[http://dx.doi.org/10.1002/chem.200400927] [PMID: 15565727]

[58]   S. Liu, Z. Zhang, and M. Han, "Gram-scale synthesis and biofunctionalization of silica-coated silver nanoparticles for fast colorimetric DNA detection", *Anal. Chem.,* vol. 77, no. 8, pp. 2595-2600, 2005.
[http://dx.doi.org/10.1021/ac0482864] [PMID: 15828798]

[59]   D. Cheng, and Q-H. Xu, "Separation distance dependent fluorescence enhancement of fluorescein isothiocyanate by silver nanoparticles", *Chem. Commun. (Camb.),* no. 3, pp. 248-250, 2007.
[http://dx.doi.org/10.1039/B612401A] [PMID: 17299628]

[60]   G. Sharma, J-S. Nam, A.R. Sharma, and S-S. Lee, "Antimicrobial potential of silver nanoparticles synthesized using medicinal herb coptidis rhizome", *Molecules,* vol. 23, no. 2268, pp. 1-12, 2018.

[61]   H Li, W. Tabis, and Y. Tang, "Hole pocket driven superconductivity and its universal features in the electron doped cuprates", *Sci. Adv,* no. eaap7349, pp. 1-7, 2019.

[62]   E. Alzahrani, and R.A. Ahmed, "Synthesis of copper nanoparticles with various sizes and shapes: application as a superior non-enzymatic sensor and antibacterial agent", *Int. J. Electrochem. Sci.,* vol. 11, pp. 4712-4723, 2016.
[http://dx.doi.org/10.20964/2016.06.83]

[63]   L. Tang, L. Zhu, F. Tang, C. Yao, J. Wang, and L. Li, "Mild synthesis of cooper nanoparticles with enhanced oxidative stabilityand their a pplication in antibacterial films", *Langmuir,* pp. 1-5, 2018.

[64]   R. Massart, "Preparation of aqueous magnetic liquids in alkaline and acidic media", *IEEE Trans. Magn.,* pp. 1247-1248, 1981.
[http://dx.doi.org/10.1109/TMAG.1981.1061188]

[65]   B-R. Lin, C-H. Chen, S. Kunuku, T-Y. Chen, T-Y. Hsiao, H. Niu, and C-P. Lee, "Fe doped magnetic nanodiamonds made by ion implantation as contrast agent for MRI, scientific reports", *Nature,* vol. 8, no. 7058, pp. 1-6, 2018.

[66]   V. Leso, and I. Iavicoli, "Palladium nanoparticles: toxicological effects and potential implications for occupational risk assessment", *Int J Mol Sci,* vol. 19, no. 2, p. 503, 2018.

[67]   A.C. Mohana, and R. Bb, "Preparation of zinc oxide nanoparticles and its characterization using scanning electron microscopy (SEM) and X-Ray diffraction (XRD)", *Procedia Technology,* vol. 24, pp. 761-766, 2016.
[http://dx.doi.org/10.1016/j.protcy.2016.05.078]

[68]   P.A. Rodnyi, and I.V. Khodyuk, "Optical and luminescence properties of zinc oxide", *Opt. Spectrosc.,* vol. 111, no. 5, pp. 776-785, 2011.
[http://dx.doi.org/10.1134/S0030400X11120216]

[69]   G. Meenakshi, and A. Sivasamy, "Synthesis and characterization of zinc oxide nanorods and its photocatalytic activities towards degradation of 2,4-D", *Ecotoxicol. Environ. Saf.,* vol. 135, pp. 243-251, 2017.
[http://dx.doi.org/10.1016/j.ecoenv.2016.10.010] [PMID: 27744194]

[70]   J. Kim, A. Dutta, B. Memarzadeh, A.V. Kildishev, H. Mosallaei, and A. Boltasseva, "Zinc oxide based

plasmonic multilayer resonator: localized and gap surface plasmon in the infrared", *ACS Photonics,* vol. 2, no. 8, pp. 1224-1230, 2015.
[http://dx.doi.org/10.1021/acsphotonics.5b00318]

[71]   J. Chen, B. Wiley, Z.Y. Li, D. Campbell, F. Saeki, H. Cang, L. Au, J. Lee, X. Li, and Y. Xia, "Gold nanocages: Engieneering their structure for biomedical applications", *Adv. Mater.,* vol. 17, pp. 2255-2261, 2005.
[http://dx.doi.org/10.1002/adma.200500833]

[72]   Y-C. Wang, É. Rhéaume, F. Lesage, and A. Kakkar, "Synthetic methodologies to gold nanoshells: an overview", *Molecules,* vol. 23, no. 11, pp. 1-28, 2018.
[http://dx.doi.org/10.3390/molecules23112851] [PMID: 30400168]

[73]   S.K.L. Maus, M. Zanella, B. Pelaez, Q. Zhang, W.J. Parak, P. del Pino, and W.J. Parak, "Inorganic core–shell nanoparticles, reference module in materials science and materials engineering", *Comprehensive Nanoscience and Technology,* vol. 1, pp. 271-287, 2011.

[74]   J. Zhang, M. Wang, and T.J. Webster, "Silver-coated gold nanorods as a promising antimicrobial agent in the treatment of cancer-related infections", *Int. J. Nanomedicine,* vol. 13, pp. 6575-6583, 2018.
[http://dx.doi.org/10.2147/IJN.S169489] [PMID: 30410338]

[75]   A. Pajor-Świerzy, D. Gaweł, E. Drzymała, R. Socha, M. Parlińska-Wojtan, K. Szczepanowicz, and P. Warszyński, "The optimization of methods of synthesis of nickel-silver core-shell nanoparticles for conductive materials", *Nanotechnology,* vol. 30, no. 1, p. 015601, 2019.
[http://dx.doi.org/10.1088/1361-6528/aae677] [PMID: 30359329]

[76]   G. Schmidt, M. Müller, P. Veit, S. Metzner, F. Bertram, J. Hartmann, H. Zhou, H-H. Wehmann, A. Waag, and J. Christen, "Direct imaging of Indium-rich triangular nanoprisms selforganized formed at the edges of InGaN/GaN core-shell nanorods", *Sci. Rep.,* vol. 8, no. 1626, pp. 1-8, 2018.

[77]   T. Chen, S. Yang, J. Chai, Y. Song, J. Fan, B. Rao, H. Sheng, H. Yu, and M. Zhu, "Crystallization-induced emission enhancement: A novel fluorescent Au-Ag bimetallic nanocluster with precise atomic structure", *Sci. Adv.,* vol. 3, no. 8, p. e1700956, 2017.
[http://dx.doi.org/10.1126/sciadv.1700956] [PMID: 28835926]

[78]   P. Xiao, J. Huang, and Y. Yu, "Recent developments in tandem white organic light-emitting diodes", *Molecules,* vol. 24, no. 151, pp. 1-28, 2019.

[79]   A.M. Eremenko, N.P. Smirnova, L.P. Mukha, and H.R. Yashan, "Silver and Gold Nanoparticles in Silica Matrices: synthesis, properties and application", *Theor. Exp. Chem.,* vol. 46, no. 2, pp. 65-88, 2010.
[http://dx.doi.org/10.1007/s11237-010-9122-5]

[80]   C. B. Cooper, I. D. Joshipura, D. P. Parakh, J. Norkett, and R. Mailen, "Thoughening stretchable fibers via serial fracturing of a metallic core", *Sci. Adv,* vol. 5, no. eaat4600, pp. 1-8, 2019.

[81]   Y-T. Tseng, Y-J. Chuang, Y-C. Wu, C-S. Yang, M-C. Wang, and F-G. Tseng, "A gold-nanoparticl--enhanced immune sensor based on fiber optic interferometry", *Nanotechnology,* vol. 19, no. 34, p. 345501, 2008.
[http://dx.doi.org/10.1088/0957-4484/19/34/345501] [PMID: 21730648]

[82]   J.L. Vivero-Escoto, and Y-T. Huang, "Inorganic-organic hybrid nanomaterials for therapeutic and diagnostic imaging applications", *Int. J. Mol. Sci.,* vol. 12, no. 6, pp. 3888-3927, 2011.
[http://dx.doi.org/10.3390/ijms12063888] [PMID: 21747714]

[83]   B. Sierra-Martin, and A. Fernandez-Barbero, "Inorganic/polymer hybrid nanoparticles for sensing applications", *Adv. Colloid Interface Sci.,* vol. 233, pp. 25-37, 2016.
[http://dx.doi.org/10.1016/j.cis.2015.12.001] [PMID: 26782148]

[84]   A.G. Bracamonte, D. Brouard, M. Lessard-Viger, D. Boudreau, and A.V. Veglia, "Nano-supramolecular complex synthesis: switch on/off enhanced fluorescence control an molecular release using a simple chemistry reaction", *Microchem. J.,* vol. 128, pp. 297-304, 2016.

[http://dx.doi.org/10.1016/j.microc.2016.05.009]

[85]   H. Izawa, K. Kawakami, M. Sumita, Y. Tateyama, J.P. Hill, and K. Ariga, "β-Cyclodextri-
        -crosslinked alginate gel for patient-controlled drug delivery systems: regulation of host-guest
        interactions with mechanical stimuli", *J. Mater. Chem. B Mater. Biol. Med.,* vol. 1, no. 16, pp. 2155-
        2161, 2013.
        [http://dx.doi.org/10.1039/c3tb00503h] [PMID: 32260848]

[86]   K. Ariga, K. Kawakami, and J. P. Hill, "Emerging pressure-release materials for drug delivery", *Exp.
        Opin. Drug Deliv,* vol. 171, no. 10, pp. 1465-1469, 2013.
        [http://dx.doi.org/10.1517/17425247.2013.819340]

[87]   A. Valizadeh, H. Mikaeli, M. SamieI, S. M. Farkhani, N. Zarghami, M. Kouhi, and A. Akbarzadeh,
        "Quantum dots: synthesis, bioapplications, and toxicity", *Nanoscale Res. Lett,* vol. 7, no. 480, pp. 1-
        14, 2012.

[88]   K.M. Goodfellow, C. Chakraborty, R. Beams, L. Novotny, and A.N. Vamivakas, "Direct on-chip
        optical plasmon detection with an atomically thin semiconductor", *Nano Lett.,* vol. 15, no. 8, pp. 5477-
        5481, 2015.
        [http://dx.doi.org/10.1021/acs.nanolett.5b01898] [PMID: 26120877]

[89]   J. A. Cardenas, S. Upshaw, N. X. Williams, M. J. Catenacci, B. J. Wiley, and A. D. Franklin, "Impact
        of morphology on printed contact performance in carbon nanotube thin-film transistors", *Adv. Funct.
        Mater,* vol. 1805727, pp. 1-7, 2018.

[90]   J-H. Kim, S.R. Kim, H.J. Kil, Y.C. Kim, and J.W. Park, "Highly conformable, transparent electrodes
        for epidermal electronics", *Nano Lett.,* vol. 18, no. 7, pp. 4531-4540, 2018.
        [http://dx.doi.org/10.1021/acs.nanolett.8b01743] [PMID: 29923729]

[91]   W. Lee, S. Kobashi, M. Nagase, Y. Jimbo, I. Saito, Y. Inoue, T. Yambe, M. Sekino, G. G. Malliaras,
        T. Yokota, M. Tanaka, and T. Someya, "Nonthrombogenic, stretchable, active multielectrode array for
        elctroanatomical mapping", *Sci. Adv,* vol. 4, no. eaau2426, pp. 1-7, 2018.

[92]   K. Sim, Z. Rao, H.-J. Kim, A. Thukral, H. Shim, and C. Yu, "Fully rubbery integrated electronics from
        high effective mobility intrinsically stretchable semiconductors", *Sci. Adv,* vol. 5, no. eaav5749, pp. 1-
        10, 2019.

[93]   M. Kanzaki, Y. Kawaguchi, and H. Kawasaki, "Fabrication of conductive copper films on flexible
        polymer substrates by low-temperature sintering of composite cu ink in air", *ACS Appl. Mater.
        Interfaces,* vol. 9, no. 24, pp. 20852-20858, 2017.
        [http://dx.doi.org/10.1021/acsami.7b04641] [PMID: 28574247]

[94]   Z. Yin, M. Jian, C. Wang, K. Xia, Z. Liu, Q. Wang, M. Zhang, H. Wang, X. Liang, X. Liang, Y. Long,
        X. Yu, and Y. Zhang, "Splash-resistant and light-weight silk-sheathed wires for textile electronics",
        Nano Lett., vol. 18, no. 11, pp. 7085-7091, 2018.
        [http://dx.doi.org/10.1021/acs.nanolett.8b03085] [PMID: 30278140]

[95]   H. Lee, E. Kim, Y. Yee, H. Kim, J. Lee, M. Kim, H. J. Yoo, and S. Yoo, "Toward all day wearable
        health monitoring: an ultralow power, reflective organic pulse oximetry sensing patch", *Sci. Adv,* vol.
        4, no. eaas9530, pp. 1-8, 2018.

[96]   J. Zhang, T. Lan, and Y. Lu, "Molecular engineering of functional nucleic acid nanomaterials toward
        In Vivo Applications", *Adv. Healthc. Mater.,* vol. 8, no. 6, p. e1801158, 2019.
        [http://dx.doi.org/10.1002/adhm.201801158] [PMID: 30725526]

[97]   P.W.K. Rothemund, "Folding DNA to create nanoscale shapes and patterns", *Nature,* vol. 440, no.
        7082, pp. 297-302, 2006.
        [http://dx.doi.org/10.1038/nature04586] [PMID: 16541064]

[98]   Y. C. Hung, D. M. Bauer, I. Ahmed, and L. Fruk, "DNA from natural sources in design of functional
        devices", *Methods,* vol. 67, no. 2, pp. 105-115, 2014.

[99]   T. Singh, N.S. Sariciftci, and G. James, "Grote, Bio-organic optoelectronic devices using DNA", *Adv.*

Polym. Sci., vol. 223, no. 1, pp. 189-212, 2010.

[100]   H.T. Maune, S-P. Han, R.D. Barish, M. Bockrath, W.A. Goddard III, P.W.K. Rothemund, and E. Winfree, "Self-assembly of carbon nanotubes into two-dimensional geometries using DNA origami templates", *Nat. Nanotechnol.,* vol. 5, no. 1, pp. 61-66, 2010.
[http://dx.doi.org/10.1038/nnano.2009.311] [PMID: 19898497]

[101]   L. Zhang, X. Zhong, E. Pavlica, S. Li, A. Klekachev, G. Bratina, T. W. Ebbesen, E. Orgiu, and P. Samori, "A nanomesh scaffold for supramolecular nanowire optoelectronic devices", *Nature nanotech,* vol. 125, pp. 1-8, 2016.

[102]   C. Wang, S. Tadepalli, J. Luan, K-K. Liu, J.J. Morrissey, E.D. Kharasch, R.R. Naik, and S. Singamaneni, "Metal-organic framework as a protective coating for biodiagnostic chips", *Adv. Mater.,* vol. 29, no. 7, pp. 1-14, 2017.
[http://dx.doi.org/10.1002/adma.201604433] [PMID: 27925296]

[103]   A. Halder, S. Karak, M. Addicoat, S. Bera, A. Chakraborty, S.H. Kunjattu, P. Pachfule, T. Heine, and R. Banerjee, "Ultrastable imine-based covalent organic frameworks for sulfuric acid recovery: an effect of interlayer hydrogen bonding", *Angew. Chem. Int. Ed. Engl.,* vol. 57, no. 20, pp. 5797-5802, 2018.
[http://dx.doi.org/10.1002/anie.201802220] [PMID: 29573097]

[104]   J. Markus, "Secondary building units as the turning point in the development of the reticular chemistry of MOFs", *Sci. Adv,* vol. 4, no. eaat9180, pp. 1-16, 2018.

[105]   N. Meinzer, W.L. Barnes, and I.R. Hooper, "Plasmonic meta-atoms and Metasurfaces", *Nat. Photonics,* vol. 8, pp. 889-898, 2014.
[http://dx.doi.org/10.1038/nphoton.2014.247]

[106]   N. Talebi, "Electronsinteracting with metamaterials:fromfew-photon sourcestoelectronoptics", *10.1117/2.1201705.006891, SPIE Newsroom,* pp. 1-3, 2017.

[107]   W. Chen, M. Tymchenko, P. Gopalan, X. Ye, Y. Wu, M. Zhang, C.B. Murray, A. Alu, and C.R. Kagan, "Large-area nanoimprinted colloidal au nanocrystal-based nanoantennas for ultrathin polarizing plasmonic metasurfaces", *Nano Lett.,* vol. 15, no. 8, pp. 5254-5260, 2015.
[http://dx.doi.org/10.1021/acs.nanolett.5b02647] [PMID: 26161503]

[108]   G.M. Mangalgiri, P. Manley, W. Riedel, and M. Schmid, "Dielectric nanorod scattering and its influence on material interfaces", *Sci. Rep.,* vol. 7, no. 1, p. 4311, 2017.
[http://dx.doi.org/10.1038/s41598-017-03721-w] [PMID: 28655917]

[109]   F. Li, H. Hou, J. Yin, and X. Jiang, "Near-infrared light responsive dynamic wrinkle patterns", *Sci Adv,* vol. 4, no. eaar5762, pp. 1-8, 2018.

[110]   N.J. Greenfield, "Using circular dichroism spectra to estimate protein secondary structure", *Nat. Protoc.,* vol. 1, no. 6, pp. 2876-2890, 2006.
[http://dx.doi.org/10.1038/nprot.2006.202] [PMID: 17406547]

[111]   Y. Tang, and A.E. Cohen, "Optical chirality and its interaction with matter", *Phys. Rev. Lett.,* vol. 104, no. 16, p. 163901, 2010.
[http://dx.doi.org/10.1103/PhysRevLett.104.163901] [PMID: 20482049]

[112]   I. Tinoco, and D.H. Turner, "Fluorescence detected circular dichroism", *Theory J Am Chem Soc,* vol. 98, pp. 6453-6456, 1976.
[http://dx.doi.org/10.1021/ja00437a003]

[113]   D.H. Turner, "Fluorescence-detected circular dichroism", *Methods Enzymol.,* vol. 49, pp. 199-214, 1978.
[http://dx.doi.org/10.1016/S0076-6879(78)49010-X] [PMID: 651663]

[114]   C. Wu1, N. Arju, G. Kelp, J.A. Fan, and J. Dominguez, "Spectrally selective chiral silicon metasurfaces based on infrared Fano resonances", *Nat. Commun.,* vol. 5, no. 3892, pp. 1-9, 2014.

[115] S. Haxha, F. AbdelMalek, F. Ouerghi, M.D.B. Charlton, A. Aggoun, and X. Fang, "Metamaterial superlenses operating at visible wavelength for imaging applications, scientific reports", *Nature,* vol. 8, no. 16119, pp. 1-15, 2018.

[116] J. Li, S. Kamin, G. Zheng, F. Neubrech, S. Zhang, and N. Liu, "Addressable metasurfaces for dynamic holography and optical information encryption", *Sci. Adv,* vol. 4, no. eaar6768, pp. 1-7, 2018.

[117] S. Tae Park, M. Lin, and A.H. Zewail, "Photon-induced near-field electron microscopy (PINEM): theoretical and experimental", *New J. Phys.,* vol. 12, no. 123028, pp. 1-57, 2010.

[118] T. Lewi, N.A. Butakov, and J.A. Schuller, "Thermal tuning capabilities of semiconductor metasurface resonators", *Nanophotonics,* vol. 8, no. 2, pp. 331-338, 2019.
[http://dx.doi.org/10.1515/nanoph-2018-0178]

[119] K. Park, J.H. Kang, X. Liu, and J. Scott, "Dynamic thermal emission control with InAs-based plasmonic metasurfaces", *Sci Adv,* vol. 4, no. eaat3163, pp. 1-7, 2018.

[120] J. Bauer, "Fabricating lightweight and ultrastrong mechanical metamaterial", *SPIE Newsroom,* vol. 1-2, 2016.
[http://dx.doi.org/10.1117/2.120173.006832]

[121] X. Ning, X. Yu, H. Wang, R. Sun, R. E. Corman, H. Li, and C. Mi Lee, "Mehanically active materials in three dimensional mesostructures", *Sci. Adv,* vol. 4, no. eaa8313, pp. 1-13, 2018.

[122] R.L. McGinnis, K. Reimund, J. Ren, L. Xia, M.R. Chowdhury, X. Sun, M. Abril, J.D. Moon, M.M. Merrick, J. Park, K.A. Stevens, J.R. McCutcheon, and B.D. Freeman, "Large-scale polymeric carbon nanotube membranes with sub-1.27-nm pores", *Sci. Adv.,* vol. 4, no. 3, p. e1700938, 2018.
[http://dx.doi.org/10.1126/sciadv.1700938] [PMID: 29536038]

[123] H. Zhang, X. Guo, J. Wu, D. Fang, and Y. Zhang, "Soft mechanical metamaterials with unusual swelling behaviour and tunable stress strain curves", *Sci. Adv,* vol. 4, no. eaar8535, pp. 1-10, 2018.

CHAPTER 4

Classical and Non-Classical Light Generation within the Near Field

Abstract: The development of varied wavelength emissions of classical light could be obtained using different materials. From the interaction of these nanomaterials within the near field of electromagnetic fields generated from metallic nanostructures, their emission could be developed and enhanced by the correctly overlapping of spectroscopical properties of both parts of the nano- or micro-luminescent device. In this way, the generation of plasmonic and enhanced plasmonics for the application of luminescence phenomena and quantum emissions was discussed.

Keywords: Classical and non-classical state of light, Enhanced plasmonics, Enhanced quantum emitters, Fluorescence resonance energy transfer (FRET), FRET coupled to plasmonics, FRET-MEF coupling, Metal enhanced fluorescence (MEF), Plasmonics.

1. PLASMONICS (P) AND ENHANCED PLASMONICS (EP)

Metallic surfaces could generate high-energy electromagnetic fields from the electronic oscillation of the surface by appropriate laser excitation. These high-energy electromagnetic fields were produced from metallic surfaces, metallic nano-patterned surfaces and metallic nanoparticles within the near field. The "near field" was defined as the electromagnetic field intensities generated within the interval of lengths below 100.0 nm, from where higher and variable intensities were measured depending on metal size and shape. The intensity showed a dependency with the distance (d) from the metallic surface of 1/d [1]. Thus, from a theoretical calculation based on the Mie theory [2] for gold nanoparticles, higher intensities were recorded below 10.0 [3], whereas the highest was found below 2.0 nm, where the electro-quantic interactions and their descriptions contributed considerably [4].

This absorption of energy from the electron of the metallic surface could be recorded from absorption measurements by spectrophotometry within colloidal dispersion and light dispersibility by dark field spectroscopy from nano-patterned surfaces [5]. Accordingly, this absorption of energy was referred to as plasmon.

This plasmonic phenomenon was observed early by E. M. Purcell *et al.* from Harvard University studying metallic particles within an electric resonant circuit that generated spontaneously high-energy radio frequencies [6]. Then these studies were extended to other particles, dimensions, materials and optical setups.

In this way, the plasmonic properties within the nanoscale showed varied absorption wavelengths depending on the intrinsic properties, size and shape [7] of the material [8]. For example aluminium, indium oxide nanoparticles showed plasmonic properties within the UV region [9], spherical silver nanoparticles with bands of absorption around 400.0 nm [10] and spherical gold nanoparticles within 510.0-550.0 nm interval, while for their nanorods, different bands were recorded within the NIR region according to material and dimension [11]. However, on the basis of their electronic properties, silver nanoparticles showed stronger plasmons than gold nanoparticles. Yet, their antifungal properties [12] and fast digestion in the presence of chloride ions [13] could affect biointeractions depending on the targeted application. Gold nanoparticles, on the other hand, showed acceptable plasmonic intensities accompanied by biocompatible properties that could be highly desired for bioapplications and nanomedicine. With these two nanomaterials only, it could be shown that different aspects form their properties in view of specific needs.

In addition, the plasmonic properties could interact with the surrounding media, which in the presence of other metallic nanostructures, generated resonant plasmons together with increased intensities between the optical resonators at short lengths within the nanoscale. This phenomenon was named enhanced plasmonics (**EP**), which could also be theoretically calculated. For example, for silver nanoparticles deposed over silica surfaces, standard plasmonic intensities were recorded, while for nanoarrays with accurate control of spacers between them, higher plasmonic emissions [14] were observed. Hence, from the inter-metallic nanoparticle interactions, enhanced plasmonic properties were found based on resonant electromagnetic fields, not explained just from the sum of the individual plasmonic nanoparticles.

Finally, in order to know/define/establish the strength of their electromagnetic field energies generated within nanoarrays, it should be mentioned based on gold 60 nanorods arrays the bacteria trapping between free spaces of nano-patterned structures The application of enhanced electromagnetic field based on **EP** at silica/silver interfaces also allowed selective intracellular surface enhanced Raman scattering detection (**SERS**) [16] and self-assembly of DNA origami honeycomb two-dimensional lattices and plasmonic metamaterials for new DNA nanotechnologies [17].

2. METAL ENHANCED FLUORESCENCE (MEF)

From the interaction of the high-energy electromagnetic fields generated from metallic surfaces and fluorophores within the near field, enhanced emissions known as metal enhanced fluorescence (**MEF**) [18, 19] were recorded. These phenomena were explained by an increased absorption and higher electronic occupancy of the excited state, leading to enhanced emission with shortened fluorescence lifetime decays [20] and diminished photobleaching properties [21].

In order to quantify these phenomena, different strategies and experiment designs were made by the deposition or incorporation of fluorescent emitters over modified metallic surfaces by colloidal nanoparticle depositions [22] or metallic nanoplatforms such as core-shell nanoarchitectures [23, 24], respectively. These systems showed enhanced emissions as compared to non-modified surfaces or metallic-less nanoarchitectures. And from the ratio of the emissions recorded in the presence and absence of metal, it was possible to determine **MEF** enhancement factors (**MEF$_{EF}$**) (Fig. **1**). In this way, different **MEF$_{EF}$** were obtained depending on metallic nanomaterials, nanoarchitectures, spatial and geometrical factors, fluorescent emitters applied and concentrations, excitation wavelengths and plasmonic coupling and the participation of other plasmonic phenomena as well as coupled energy transfer processes.

Consequently, stronger plasmon from silver nanostructures showed greater improvements than other metals applied, due to their intrinsic electronic properties [25].

High dependency on improvements with spacer lengths between the fluorescent emitter and the metallic surfaces was also reported. Shorter spacer lengths within the near field beyond 10.0 nm showed higher enhancement while longer spacer lengths diminished/decreased values [23]. However, when the fluorophore was placed close to the metallic surface, a quenching effect was observed [26].

Then, in relation to spatial and geometrical factors, it is important to mention the relative position of the fluorophore within the electromagnetic field [27] and the orientation of the dipole moments [28], as well as the quantum yields of the fluorescent emitters. In general, lower quantum yields (QY) showed higher improvement for standard fluorophores [29]; however, high improvement for quantum-dots with higher (QY) [30] was also shown. Therefore, variable enhancement could be recorded according to the fluorophore and metal applied.

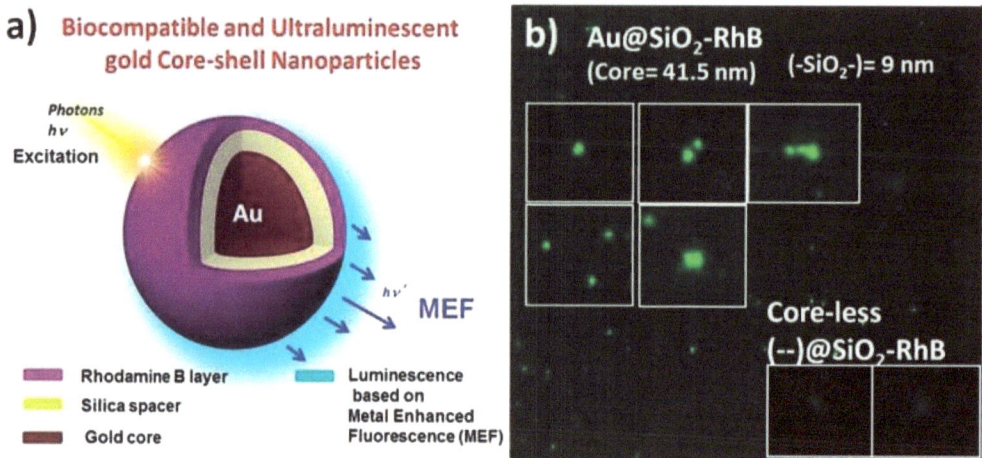

Fig. (1). a) Scheme of biocompatible and ultraluminescent gold core-shell nanoparticles (Au@SiO$_2$-RhB) modified with Rhodamine B (RhB) based on metal enhanced fluorescence (MEF).b) Laser fluorescence microscopy of Au@SiO$_2$–RhB nanoparticles with a silica spacer length of 9-10 nm and inset images of core-less (--)@SiO$_2$-RhB [24].

It should also be noted that the **MEF** effect was not just an effect of enhanced scattering of light. This could be demonstrated in the design of silica nanocomposites with incorporation of different concentrations of fluorophores and metallic nanoparticles [31]. And, hence, it was demonstrated that only in the presence of the correct plasmonic tuning of the nanostructures accompanied with right plasmon and fluorophore excitation, it was achieved to couple the high-energy electromagnetic field from the metallic surface and the fluorophore excitation. Other plasmonic phenomena related with inter-nanoparticle interactions or interactions of metallic surfaces could also be reported, such as enhanced plasmonics (**EP**) from individual dimmers [32, 33] or trimmers and highly controlled nanoaggregates [34] to nanoarrays and nano-patterned surfaces [35] and optical resonators [36, 37] from hollowed metallic nanostructures [38] that could greatly affect the emissions of fluorophores within the near fields.

3. FLUORESCENCE RESONANCE ENERGY TRANSFER (FRET)

Numerous studies have been published discussing the mechanisms of excited electronic energies transfer, based on well separated atomic or molecular electronic systems such as the simplest case of two distinct atoms within a confined space by T. Forster [39] to inter-molecular transfers within complex matrixes [40] and new advanced applied developments of microdevices [41].

Fluorescence resonance energy transfer (**FRET**) from a donor/acceptor pair of energy was shown to be highly and mostly dependent on the inter-emitter and acceptor spacer lengths (R). Linked to this parameter, the Forster distance (R_0) of resonant energy pairs [42] should also be discussed. The (R_0) was defined as the distance between the donor and acceptor, where the energy transfer efficiency was 50%. For optimal **FRET**, donor emission and acceptor absorption should overlap, with a decreased overlapping between both absorption and emissions of the donor/acceptor pair.

Moreover, from single molecule detection (**SMD**) by fluorescence microscopy, an influence of the relative fluorophore orientation, their separation diffusion of and quenching effect [43] (Fig. **2**) was found. This study of **SMD** showed the importance and high sensitivity within the molecular dimensions and nanoscale lengths. As reported previously in the literature, with donor/acceptor lengths shorter than 1.0 nm, quenching by homo-transfer was reported. On the other hand, with lengths within 2-10 nm interval of distances, energy transfers were successfully recorded from fluorescent organic emitters and quantum emitter particles [44].

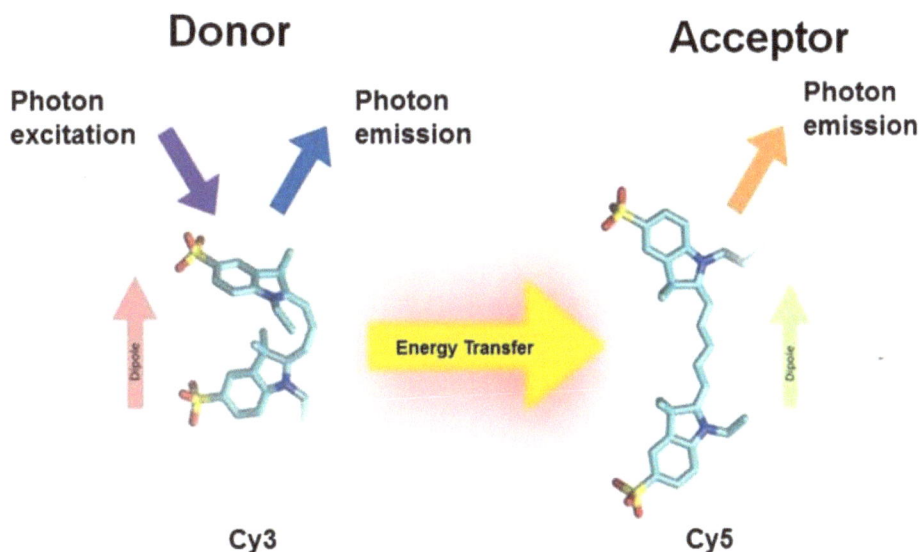

Fig. (2). Single-molecule FRET event. A FRET event starts when a molecule labelled by a donor/acceptor pair diffuses into a volume of sufficiently large laser intensity near the focal point (left). The counts for detected photon emissions for the acceptor nA and donor nD are recorded until the molecule diffuses out of the focal volume (top right). During the donor excitation either a photon is emitted or energy is non-radiatively transferred to the acceptor and emitted with rates that depend on the molecular conformation (lower right) [43].

This phenomenon has allowed not only fluorescence energy resonance, but also optical resonators with lasing properties based on π-conjugated organic microcrystals by the right tuning of materials [45]. Additionally, due to the high sensitivity of this phenomenon, many applications have been reported in relation to biomolecular interactions and 3D biostructures, as well as new synthetic approaches in nanotechnology and biotechnology.

At the same time, current advances in fluorescence microscopy, in addition to the development of new fluorescent probes, have turned fluorescence resonance energy transfer (**FRET**) a powerful technique for studying molecular interactions inside living cells with improved spatial (angstrom) and temporal (nanosecond) resolution, distance range and sensitivity and a broader range of biological applications [46]. As an example, screening for protein-protein interactions by fluorescence lifetime imaging microscopy (**FLIM**) [47] has allowed accurate relative   localization   between   these   biostructures   within   cells. Besides   the application of synthetic fluorescent labellers, bioluminescent proteins have been used as centers of energy for energy transfer [48] and bioimaging [49].

Moreover, increasing interest in RNA technology has led to the production/design of different RNA nanoarchitectures as potential therapeutic agents [50, 51] and to the development of a genetically encodable **FRET** system using fluorescent RNA aptamers [52]. Similarly, DNA origamis are potential synthetic biostructures for the design of **FRET** systems [53].

Recently, by comparing small-angle x-ray scattering (SAXS) and **FRET** experiments of unfolded proteins in water *versus* chemical denaturant conditions [54], protein compaction has not been observed. This observation has a high impact and implications in relation to bioapplications.

Moreover, **FRET** was used for designing synthetic molecular **FRET** systems [55] and synthetic nanoarchitectures for targeted applications, including self-assembled nanoscale biosensors based on quantum dot **FRET** donors [56], synthetic confined donor/acceptor pairs coupled to bioreactions within nanoparticles [57] and **FRET** fluorescent nanoparticles based on a microporous organic polymers [58].

However, even if **FRET**, **RET** or other energy transfer processes were considered as short range phenomena (**FRET** dependency with $R \sim 1/R^6$), a recent study it was reported about long-distance operator for a nanophotonic energy transfer based on a confined nanocavity formed by two silver mirrors that supported an electromagnetic mode which matched with the donor/acceptor incorporated within these Nanocavities [59]. Thus, this long-distance operator for energy transfer nanophotonics can be used to enhance the electromagnetic coupling between molecules. The short range of **FRET** results from the small interaction between visible light (a photon) and matter (an exciton) in vacuum. However, this coupling can be increased (or decreased) if the photonic environment of the exciton is modified. For example, when a molecule is located inside a cavity able to confine electromagnetic (EM) fields, the light-matter interaction is enhanced. In such systems, two different regimes of light-matter coupling can be found.

In energy transduction within micro- and nanodevices, new modes of energy transfer should be taken into account. Further considerations are discussed in the section of waveguide signaling.

4. COUPLED PHENOMENA (P-FRET; MEF-FRET; EP-MEF)

As discussed in the previous sections, from the interaction of the electromagnetic fields within the near field with different types of emitters, new properties were generated. In this way, the emissions were increased along with shortened fluorescence lifetime decays. Similarly, the interaction of the light emitted by a **FRET** pathway coupled to metallic surfaces showed enhanced emissions from the donor/acceptor pair as compared to individual emitters [60]. This enhanced Forster resonance energy transfer on particles showed dependency on donor/acceptor distance, excitation wavelength [61], size of nanoparticles and distance from the metallic surfaces [62]. In addition, from **FRET-MEF** coupling, with emissions even higher than only in the presence of **MEF** phenomenon [63] was observed.

This effect was observed by static fluorescence, single nanoparticle analysis by laser fluorescence microscopy and in flow cytometry (**IFC**) coupled to optical setups for enhanced resolution of nanoparticles. In this issue, the importance of the control of the nanoarchitecture dimensions should be particularly underlined in order to analyze the previously discussed variables that affected both phenomena [64].

To enhance emissions based on plasmonic phenomena, **MEF** could be applied with enhanced plasmonic (**EP**) nanostructures. In the previous section, we have already discussed the way in which **EP** could generate enhanced high-energy electromagnetic fields that could interact with fluorophores in the near surrounding of the **EP** metallic nanosurfaces. Consequently, research has shown that different nanoarchitectures and nanoarrays with **EP** plasmonic properties could be used for potential **MEF** applications. However, although many theoretical calculations have been reported, it was not the case of experimental studies. A case in point is the feasibility of using bimetallic plasmonic nanostructures to enhance the intrinsic emission of biomolecules as proteins with bimetallic nanostructures made of silver (Ag) and aluminum (Al) to implement **MEF** phenomenon for improving the intrinsic emission in the ultraviolet (UV) spectral region. The fluorescence intensity and lifetime of a tryptophan analogue N-acetyl-L-tryptophanamide (NATA) and a tyrosine analogue nacetyl-L-tyro sinamide (NATA-tyr) [65] were evaluated. The increase in fluorescence intensity of up to 10-fold and consequent decrease in the lifetime of aminoacids were recorded in the presence of bimetallic nanostructures when compared to quartz controls. The model of protein assay consisted of biotinylated bovine serum albumin (bt-BSA) and streptavidin on bimetallic nanostructured substrates to investigate distance-dependent effects on the extent of **MEF** from bimetallic nanostructures. A maximum improvement of over 15-fold for two layers of bt-BSA and streptavidin was recorded. These improvements were explained by finite-difference time domain (FDTD) calculations. While on the other hand, different approaches have been studied, such as metal-enhanced single-molecule fluorescence on silver particle monomer and dimer coupling effects between metal particles to gain insights into molecular detection [66]. In addition, the coupling of emission to nanoplasmonic resonator arrays from modified surfaces with targeted laser excitations could be also applied in biosensing based upon molecular confinement within metallic nanocavity arrays [67]. These nanocavity arrays were produced with less than half the wavelength-typically100– 200nm in diameter; e-beam lithography was used to pattern with positive resist, polymethylmethacrylate (PMMA), followed by a reactive ion *etc*hing (RIE) step (with silicon nitride used as a mask layer) to transfer the nanocavity array patterns to metal films [68].

To conclude, we could mention that all these coupled phenomena, as well as other modes of coupled signaling, could be applied to nano- and microdevices designs to detect and transduce different types of signals and to develop new imaging modes by incorporation and coupling of technological devices as smartphones and fluorescence microscopy techniques [69]. In the next sections, we will discuss these targeted designs and applications on the basis of the previous phenomena and coupled modes of signals.

5. ENHANCED QUANTUM EMITTERS

From confined electrons, new quantum properties were generated, such as lasing modes [70], quantum conductivity [71, 72] and quantum emission properties [73, 74]. The most commonly known quantum emitters comprise the quantum dots that could be obtained by synthetic methodologies in colloidal dispersions [75]. As discussed in the **MEF** section, these emissions have been even enhanced by the interaction of high electromagnetic fields from plasmonic nanoarchitectures [76]. However, this research theme has proved to be largely applied to quantum and optical micro- and nanodevices. For example, Photonic quantum teleportation could be employed with on demand solid state quantum emitters [77]. Quantum emission and teleportation could be applied to quantum communication science and technology. Hence, quantum phenomena should be encoded in photon pairs as in GaAs quantum dot networks with femtosecond laser excitation. These highly symmetric GaAs/AlGaAs quantum dots were fabricated *via* the droplet *etc*hing method [78] with 12% of quantum efficiency from the quantum surfaces obtained. It should be noted that these types of quantum signaling were guided by teleportation through fiber channels [79], opening their applications to microdevices in macroinstrumentation (Fig. **3**).

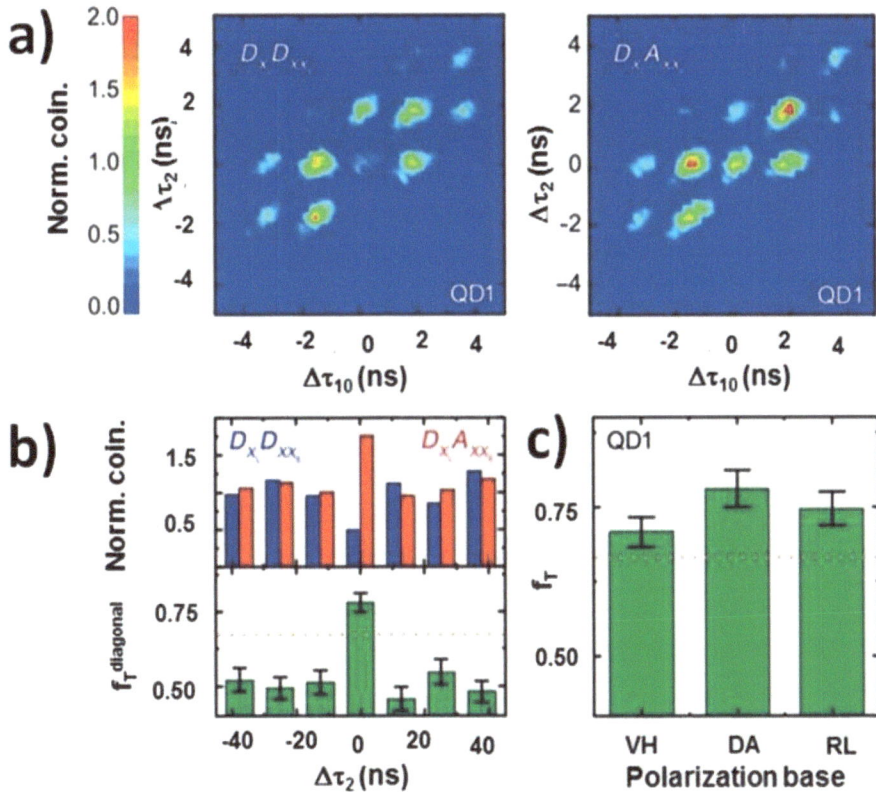

Fig. (3). a) Normalized third-order correlation of a D-polarized X input state for copolarized (left) and crosspolarized (right) detection of XX photons. b) Integrated coincidences for both detection bases for different excitation cycles (top) and the corresponding calculated teleportation fidelity (bottom). c) Teleportation fidelities for a full set of orthogonal input states. The classical limit is highlighted as a dashed orange line [77].

Quantum-optical influence on optoelectronics showed to be of high impact over the last years for future technology developments [80]. The incorporation of quantum optics in the physics and engineering of electronic components within quantum and photonic circuits showed to be particularly interesting in the fabrication of microdevices and nanodevices. Here, electrodynamics [81], as already mentioned in the plasmonic section, has assumed central importance to predict the electronic waves and interactions through materials. In this sense, the discussion of the development of low threshold lasers, when the channeling of spontaneous emission into the lasing mode becomes so efficient, and photon statistics to produce single-photon sources for applications such as quantum information processing needs to be brought up in the design of devices.

These studies also reached the level of analysis of ultrafast electron calorimetry of quantum materials by mode selective electron phonon coupling for the most promising frontiers in the quest for faster, lightweight, energy efficient technologies [82]. In all these studies, different techniques have been adopted for the fabrication of chips, and within this subject/area, there is significant knowledge that exceeds the scope of this section. However, we could highlight the uses of self-assembled monolayers (**SAM**), molecular wires, ionic liquids, semiconductor materials, silica materials and lithography techniques [83] for targeted functionalization.

CONCLUDING REMARKS

Here, it should be underlined how the coupling of different modes of electromagnetic wavelengths was achieved from metallic surfaces, molecules and quantum emitters in order to control absorptions and emissions of luminescent materials along with the complete electromagnetic field range. In this respect, we described the **MEF** based on the plasmonic and varied luminescent emitter interactions and on enhanced plasmonic phenomena. We have also discussed **FRET** coupled to plasmonic and enhanced plasmonics as well as **MEF**. It was finally referred to the enhancement of these phenomena at quantum emission levels with potential applications not only in luminescent devices but also in quantum circuits.

REFERENCES

[1]   M.L. Viger, L.S. Live, O.D. Therrien, and D. Boudreau, "Reduction of self-quenching in fluorescent silica-coated silver nanoparticles", *Plasmonics,* vol. 3, pp. 33-40, 2008.
[http://dx.doi.org/10.1007/s11468-007-9051-x]

[2]   T. Jensen, L. Kelly, A. Lazarides, and G.C. Schatz, "Electrodynamics of noble metal nanoparticles and nanoparticle clusters", *J. Cluster Sci.,* vol. 10, no. 12, pp. 295-317, 1999.
[http://dx.doi.org/10.1023/A:1021977613319]

[3]   J. Zhu, and K. Zhu, "Li-Quing Huang; using gold colloid nanoparticles to modulate the surface enhanced fluorescence of rhodamine B", *Phys. Lett. A,* vol. 372, pp. 3283-3288, 2008.
[http://dx.doi.org/10.1016/j.physleta.2008.01.067]

[4] I. Wayan Sudiarta, and D.J. Wallace Geldart, "Solving the schrödinger equation for a charged particle in a magnetic field using the finite difference time domain method", *Phys. Lett. A,* vol. 372, pp. 3145-3148, 2008.
[http://dx.doi.org/10.1016/j.physleta.2008.01.078]

[5] Z. Liu, H.H. Wang, and H. Li, "Red shift of plasmon resonance frequency due to the interacting Ag nanoparticles embedded in single crystal sio2 by implantation", *Appl. Phys. Lett.,* vol. 72, no. 15, pp. 1823-1850, 1998.
[http://dx.doi.org/10.1063/1.121196]

[6] E.M. Purcell, "Spontaneous emission probabilities at radio frequencies", *Phys. Rev.,* vol. 69, pp. 681-682, 1946.

[7] L.M. Liz-Marzán, "Tailoring surface plasmons through the morphology and assembly of metal nanoparticles", *Langmuir,* vol. 22, no. 1, pp. 32-41, 2006.
[http://dx.doi.org/10.1021/la0513353] [PMID: 16378396]

[8] S.A. Maiera, and H.A. Atwater, "Plasmonics: Localization and guiding of electromagnetic energy in metal/dielectric structures", *J. Appl. Phys.,* vol. 98, no. 011101, pp. 1-10, 2005.
[http://dx.doi.org/10.1063/1.1951057]

[9] J. Proust, S. Schuermans, J. Martin, D. Gérard, T. Maurer, and J. Plain, *Synthesis of aluminum nanoparticles for UV plasmonics, JTuA58, CLEO:2013.* Technical Digest OSA, 2013, pp. 1-2.

[10] L. Guo, A. Guan, X. Lin, C. Zhang, and G. Chen, "Preparation of a new core-shell Ag@SiO2 nanocomposite and its application for fluorescence enhancement", *Talanta,* vol. 82, no. 5, pp. 1696-1700, 2010.
[http://dx.doi.org/10.1016/j.talanta.2010.07.051] [PMID: 20875565]

[11] L.M. Liz-Marzán, "Tailoring surface plasmons through the morphology and assembly of metal nanoparticles", *Langmuir,* vol. 22, no. 1, pp. 32-41, 2006.
[http://dx.doi.org/10.1021/la0513353] [PMID: 16378396]

[12] H.H. Lara Ayala, and N.V. Núñez, "Ixtepan Turrent Ld, Rodríguez Padilla C. Bactericidal effect of silver nanoparticles against multidrug-resistant bacteria", *World J. Microbiol. Biotechnol.,* vol. 26, no. 4, pp. 615-621, 2010.
[http://dx.doi.org/10.1007/s11274-009-0211-3]

[13] "Digestion of silver in acidic ferric chloride and copper chloride solutions", *Hydrometallurgy,* vol. 20, no. 2, pp. 219-233, 1988.
[http://dx.doi.org/10.1016/0304-386X(88)90053-9]

[14] R. Luchowski, N. Calander, T. Shtoyko, E. Apicella, J. Borejdo, Z. Gryczynski, and I. Gryczynski, "Plasmonic platforms of self-assembled silver nanostructures in application to fluorescence", *J. Nanophotonics,* vol. 4, no. 043516, pp. 1-14, 2010.
[http://dx.doi.org/10.1117/1.3500463] [PMID: 21403765]

[15] M. Righini, P. Ghenuche, S. Cherukulappurath, V. Myroshnychenko, F.J. García de Abajo, and R. Quidant, "Nano-optical trapping of Rayleigh particles and Escherichia coli bacteria with resonant optical antennas", *Nano Lett.,* vol. 9, no. 10, pp. 3387-3391, 2009.
[http://dx.doi.org/10.1021/nl803677x] [PMID: 19159322]

[16] D. Radziuk, and H. Möhwald, "Surpassingly competitive electromagnetic field enhancement at the silica/silver interface for selective intracellular surface enhanced Raman scattering detection", *ACS Nano,* vol. 9, no. 3, pp. 2820-2835, 2015.
[http://dx.doi.org/10.1021/nn506741v] [PMID: 25704061]

[17] P. Wang, S. Gaitanaros, S. Lee, M. Bathe, W.M. Shih, and Y. Ke, "Programming Self-Assembly of DNA Origami Honeycomb Two-Dimensional Lattices and Plasmonic Metamaterials", *J. Am. Chem. Soc.,* vol. 138, no. 24, pp. 7733-7740, 2016.
[http://dx.doi.org/10.1021/jacs.6b03966] [PMID: 27224641]

[18]   C.D. Geddes, and J.R. Lakowicz, "Editorial. Metal-Enhanced Fluorescence", *J. Fluoresc.,* vol. 12, no. 2, pp. 121-129, 2002.
[http://dx.doi.org/10.1023/A:1016875709579]

[19]   J.R. Lakowicz, K. Ray, M. Chowdhury, H. Szmacinski, Y. Fu, J. Zhang, and K. Nowaczyk, "Plasmon-controlled fluorescence: a new paradigm in fluorescence spectroscopy", *Analyst (Lond.),* vol. 133, no. 10, pp. 1308-1346, 2008.
[http://dx.doi.org/10.1039/b802918k] [PMID: 18810279]

[20]   J.R. Lakowicz, "Radiative decay engineering 5: metal-enhanced fluorescence and plasmon emission", *Anal. Biochem.,* vol. 337, no. 2, pp. 171-194, 2005.
[http://dx.doi.org/10.1016/j.ab.2004.11.026] [PMID: 15691498]

[21]   J.R. Lakowicz, I. Gryczynski, J. Malicka, Z. Gryczynski, and C.D. Geddes, "Enhanced and localized multiphoton excited fluorescence near metallic silver islands: metallic islands can increase probe photostability", *J. Fluoresc.,* vol. 12, no. 3-4, pp. 299-302, 2002.
[http://dx.doi.org/10.1023/A:1021341305229] [PMID: 32377062]

[22]   J. Lukomska, J. Malicka, I. Gryczynski, and J.R. Lakowicz, "Fluorescence enhancements on silver colloid coated surfaces", *J. Fluoresc.,* vol. 14, no. 4, pp. 417-423, 2004.
[http://dx.doi.org/10.1023/B:JOFL.0000031823.04926.75] [PMID: 15617384]

[23]   J. Asselin, P. Legros, A. Gregoire, and D. Boudreau, "Correlating metal enhanced fluorescence and structural properties in Ag@SiO2 core-shell nanoparticles", *Plasmonics,* vol. 11, no. 5, pp. 1369-1376, 2016.
[http://dx.doi.org/10.1007/s11468-016-0186-5]

[24]   M. Rioux, D. Gontero, A.V. Veglia, A. Guillermo Bracamonte, and D. Boudreau, "Synthesis of ultraluminiscent gold core-shell nanoparticles as nanoimaging platforms for biosensing applications based on metal enhanced fluorescence", *RSC Advances,* vol. 7, pp. 10252-10258, 2017.
[http://dx.doi.org/10.1039/C6RA27649K]

[25]   K. Lance Kelly, E. Coronado, L.L. Zhao, and G.C. Schatz, "The optical properties of metal nanoparticles: the influence of size, shape, and dielectric environment", *J. Phys. Chem. B,* vol. 107, pp. 668-667, 2003.
[http://dx.doi.org/10.1021/jp026731y]

[26]   E. Dulkeith, A.C. Morteani, T. Niedereichholz, T.A. Klar, J. Feldmann, S.A. Levi, F.C. van Veggel, D.N. Reinhoudt, M. Möller, and D.I. Gittins, "Fluorescence quenching of dye molecules near gold nanoparticles: radiative and nonradiative effects", *Phys. Rev. Lett.,* vol. 89, no. 20, 2002.203002
[http://dx.doi.org/10.1103/PhysRevLett.89.203002] [PMID: 12443474]

[27]   S. Nie, and S.R. Emory, "Probing single molecules and single nanoparticles by surface-enhanced raman scattering", *Science,* vol. 275, no. 5303, pp. 1102-1106, 1997.
[http://dx.doi.org/10.1126/science.275.5303.1102] [PMID: 9027306]

[28]   A. Senes, S.C.J. Meskers, H. Greiner, K. Suzuki, H. Kaji, C. Adachi, J.S. Wilson, and R.A.J. Janssen, "Increasing the horizontal orientation of transition dipole moments in solution processed small molecular emitters", *J Mater Chem C Mater,* vol. 5, no. 26, pp. 6555-6562, 2017.
[http://dx.doi.org/10.1039/C7TC01568B] [PMID: 29308204]

[29]   A.I. Dragan, and C.D. Geddes, "Metal-enhanced fluorescence: The role of quantum yield, Q0, in enhanced fluorescence", *Appl. Phys. Lett.,* vol. 100, no. 093115, pp. 1-4, 2012.
[http://dx.doi.org/10.1063/1.3692105]

[30]   Y. Fu, J. Zhang, and J.R. Lakowicz, "Silver-enhanced fluorescence emission of single quantum dot nanocomposites", *Chem. Commun. (Camb.),* vol. 3, no. 3, pp. 313-315, 2009.
[http://dx.doi.org/10.1039/B816736B] [PMID: 19209313]

[31]   M. Martini, P. Perriat, M. Montagna, R. Pansu, C. Julien, O. Tillement, and S. Roux, "How gold particles suppress concentration quenching of fluorophores encapsulated in silica beads", *J. Phys.*

Chem. C, vol. 113, pp. 17669-17677, 2009.
[http://dx.doi.org/10.1021/jp9044572]

[32]   J. Zhang, Y. Fu, M.H. Chowdhury, and J.R. Lakowicz, "Metal-enhanced single-molecule fluorescence on silver particle monomer and dimer: coupling effect between metal particles", *Nano Lett.,* vol. 7, no. 7, pp. 2101-2107, 2007.
[http://dx.doi.org/10.1021/nl071084d] [PMID: 17580926]

[33]   C. Vietz, I. Kaminska, M. Sanz Paz, P. Tinnefeld, and G.P. Acuna, "Broadband fluorescence enhancement with self-assembled silver nanoparticle optical antennas", *ACS Nano,* vol. 11, no. 5, pp. 4969-4975, 2017.
[http://dx.doi.org/10.1021/acsnano.7b01621] [PMID: 28445644]

[34]   B. Xia, F. He, and L. Li, "Metal enhanced fluorescence using aggregated silver nanoparticles", *Colloids Surf. A Physicochem. Eng. Asp.,* vol. 444, pp. 9-14, 2014.
[http://dx.doi.org/10.1016/j.colsurfa.2013.12.029]

[35]   E.G. Matveeva, T. Shtoyko, I. Gryczynski, I. Akopova, and Z. Gryczynski, "Fluorescence quenching/enhancement surface assays: signal manipulation using silver-coated gold nanoparticles", *Chem. Phys. Lett.,* vol. 454, no. 1-3, pp. 85-90, 2008.
[http://dx.doi.org/10.1016/j.cplett.2008.01.075] [PMID: 19279673]

[36]   M. Ringler, A. Schwemer, M. Wunderlich, A. Nichtl, K. Kürzinger, T.A. Klar, and J. Feldmann, "Shaping emission spectra of fluorescent molecules with single plasmonic nanoresonators", *Phys. Rev. Lett.,* vol. 100, no. 20, 2008.203002
[http://dx.doi.org/10.1103/PhysRevLett.100.203002] [PMID: 18518528]

[37]   S. Chuan, "Optical gain in surface plasmon nanocavity oscillators", *Journal of Nanophotonics,* vol. 10, no. 1, pp. 1-11, 2016.
[http://dx.doi.org/] [PMID: 016015]

[38]   M.A. Mahmoud, D. O'Neil, and M.A. El-Sayed, "Hollow and solid metal nanostructures in sensing and in nanocatalysis", *Chem. Mater.,* vol. 26, pp. 44-58, 2014.
[http://dx.doi.org/10.1021/cm4020892]

[39]   T. Forster, "10th Spiers memorial lecture. transfer mechanisms of electronic excitation", *Discuss. Faraday Soc.,* vol. 27, pp. 7-17, 1959.
[http://dx.doi.org/10.1039/DF9592700007]

[40]   A.B. Sigalov, "Targeting intramembrane protein-protein interactions: novel therapeutic strategy of millions years old", *Adv. Protein Chem. Struct. Biol.,* vol. 111, pp. 61-99, 2018.
[http://dx.doi.org/10.1016/bs.apcsb.2017.06.004] [PMID: 29459036]

[41]   S. Kim, D. Hee Shin, J. Kim, and C.W. Jang, "S. S. Kang J. M. Kim, J. Hwan Kim, D. H. Lee, J. H. Kim, S.-H. Choi, S. W. Hwang, Energy transfer from an individual silica nanoparticle to graphene quantum dots and resulting enhancement of photodetector responsivity", *Sci. Rep.,* vol. 6, no. 27145, pp. 1-8, 2016.

[42]   H. Dacres, J. Wang, M.M. Dumancic, and S.C. Trowell, "Experimental determination of the Förster distance for two commonly used bioluminescent resonance energy transfer pairs", *Anal. Chem.,* vol. 82, no. 1, pp. 432-435, 2010.
[http://dx.doi.org/10.1021/ac9022956] [PMID: 19957970]

[43]   B. Wallace, and P. J. Atzberger, " Forster resonance energy transfer: Role of diffusion of fluorophore orientation and separation in observed shifts of FRET efficiency", *PLoS ONE,* vol. 12, no. 5, p. e0177122, 2019. 1-22

[44]   M.S. Kodaimati, C. Wang, C. Chapman, G.C. Schatz, and E.A. Weiss, "Distance-dependence of interparticle energy transfer in the near-infrared within electrostatic assemblies of pbs quantum dots", *ACS Nano,* vol. 11, no. 5, pp. 5041-5050, 2017.
[http://dx.doi.org/10.1021/acsnano.7b01778] [PMID: 28398717]

[45]   D. Okada, and S. Azzini, H. Nishioka, A. Ichimura, H. Tsuji, E. Nakamura, F. Sasaki, C. Genet, T. W. Ebbesen, Y. Yamamoto, "π Electronic cocrystal microcavities with selective vibronicmode light amplification: toward Förster resonance energy transfer lasin", *Nano Lett.,* vol. 8, no. 7, pp. 4396-4402, 2018.
[http://dx.doi.org/10.1021/acs.nanolett.8b01442] [PMID: 29902018]

[46]   R.B. Sekar, and A. Periasamy, "Fluorescence resonance energy transfer (FRET) microscopy imaging of live cell protein localizations", *J. Cell Biol.,* vol. 160, no. 5, pp. 629-633, 2003.
[http://dx.doi.org/10.1083/jcb.200210140] [PMID: 12615908]

[47]   A. Margineanu, J. Jia Chan, D.J. Kelly, S.C. Warren, D. Flatters, S. Kumar, M. Katan, C.W. Dunsby, and P.M.W. French, "Screening for protein-protein interactions using Förster resonance energy transfer (FRET) and fluorescence lifetime imaging microscopy (FLIM), Scientific Reports", *Nature,* vol. 6, no. 2818, pp. 1-16, 2016.

[48]   C. El Khamlichi, F. Reverchon-Assadi, N. Hervouet-Coste, L. Blot, E. Reiter, and S. Morisset-Lopez, "Bioluminescence resonance energy transfer as a method to study protein-protein interactions: application to G protein coupled receptor biology", *Molecules,* vol. 24, no. 3, pp. 1-21, 2019.
[http://dx.doi.org/10.3390/molecules24030537] [PMID: 30717191]

[49]   D. Paleček, P. Edlund, S. Westenhoff, and D. Zigmantas, "Quantum coherence as a witness of vibronically hot energy transfer in bacterial reaction center", *Sci. Adv.,* vol. 3, no. 9, 2017.e1603141
[http://dx.doi.org/10.1126/sciadv.1603141] [PMID: 28913419]

[50]   G.W. Gordon, G. Berry, X.H. Liang, B. Levine, and B. Herman, "Quantitative fluorescence resonance energy transfer measurements using fluorescence microscopy", *Biophys. J.,* vol. 74, no. 5, pp. 2702-2713, 1998.
[http://dx.doi.org/10.1016/S0006-3495(98)77976-7] [PMID: 9591694]

[51]   D. Shu, H. Zhang, R. Petrenko, J. Meller, and P. Guo, "Dual-channel single-molecule fluorescence resonance energy transfer to establish distance parameters for RNA nanoparticles", *ACS Nano,* vol. 4, no. 11, pp. 6843-6853, 2010.
[http://dx.doi.org/10.1021/nn1014853] [PMID: 20954698]

[52]   M.D.E. Jepsen, S.M. Sparvath, T.B. Nielsen, A.H. Langvad, G. Grossi, K.V. Gothelf, and E.S. Anderse, "Development of a genetically encodable FRET system using fluorescent RNA aptamers", *Nat. Commun.,* vol. 9, no. 18, pp. 1-10, 2018.
[http://dx.doi.org/10.1038/s41467-017-02435-x]

[53]   Y. Choi, L. Kotthoff, L. Olejko, U. Resch-Genger, and I. Bald, "DNA origami-based Förster resonance energy-transfer nanoarrays and their application as ratiometric sensors", *ACS Appl. Mater. Interfaces,* vol. 10, no. 27, pp. 23295-23302, 2018.
[http://dx.doi.org/10.1021/acsami.8b03585] [PMID: 29916243]

[54]   R. B. Best, W. Zheng, A. Borgia, K. Buholzer, M. B. Borgia, H. Hofmann, A. Soranno, D. Nettels, K. Gast, A. Grishaev, and B. Schuler, "Innovative scattering analysis shows that hydrophobic disordered proteins are expanded in water", *Science,* vol. 361, pp. 1-2, 2018.
[PMID: eaar7101]

[55]   K. Isayama, N. Aizawa, J.Y. Kim, and T. Yasuda, "Modulating photo- and electroluminescence in a stimuli-responsive π-conjugated donor-acceptor molecular system", *Angew. Chem. Int. Ed. Engl.,* vol. 57, no. 37, pp. 11982-11986, 2018.
[http://dx.doi.org/10.1002/anie.201806863] [PMID: 30039632]

[56]   I. L. Medintz, A. R. Clapp, H. Mattoussi, E. R. Goldman, B. Fisher, and J. M. Mauro, *Self-assembled nanoscale biosensors based on quantum dot FRET donors, 9LMJ 9L JA9DK,* pp. 630-638, 2003.
[http://dx.doi.org/10.1038/nmat961] [PMID: 12942071]

[57]   L. Nuhn, S. Van Herck, A. Best, K. Deswarte, M. Kokkinopoulou, I. Lieberwirth, K. Koynov, B.N. Lambrecht, and B.G. De Geest, "Forster-resonanzenergietransfer-basierter Nachweis intrazellularer Ketal-Hydrolyse in synthetisch vernetzten Nanopartikeln", *Angew. Chem.,* vol. 130, pp. 1-7, 2018.

[http://dx.doi.org/10.1002/ange.201803847]

[58]   A. Patra, J-M. Koenen, and U. Scherf, "Fluorescent nanoparticles based on a microporous organic polymer network: fabrication and efficient energy transfer to surface-bound dyes", *Chem. Commun. (Camb.)*, vol. 47, no. 34, pp. 9612-9614, 2011.
[http://dx.doi.org/10.1039/c1cc13420e] [PMID: 21805006]

[59]   F.J. Garcia-Vidal, and J. Feist, "Long-distance operator for energy transfer", *Science*, vol. 357, no. 6358, pp. 1357-1358, 2017.
[http://dx.doi.org/10.1126/science.aao4268] [PMID: 28963244]

[60]   J.R. Lakowicz, and Y. Shen, S. D"Auria, J. Malicka, J. Fang, Z. Gryczinski, I. Gryczynski, "Effects of silver islands films on fluorescence intensity, lifetimes, and resonance energy transfer", *Anal. Biochem.*, vol. 301, pp. 261-277, 2002.
[http://dx.doi.org/10.1006/abio.2001.5503] [PMID: 11814297]

[61]   J. Lee, S. Lee, M. Jen, and Y. Pang, "Metal-enhanced fluorescence: wavelength-dependent ultrafast energy transfer", *J. Phys. Chem. C*, vol. 119, pp. 23285-23291, 2015.
[http://dx.doi.org/10.1021/acs.jpcc.5b08744]

[62]   J. Zhang, Y. Fu, M.H. Chowdhury, and J.R. Lakowicz, "Enhanced förster resonance energy transfer on single metal particle. 2. dependence on donor-acceptor separation distance, particle size, and distance from metal surface", *J Phys Chem C Nanomater Interfaces*, vol. 111, no. 32, pp. 11784-11792, 2007.
[http://dx.doi.org/10.1021/jp067887r] [PMID: 19890406]

[63]   M. Lessard-Viger, D. Brouard, and D. Boudreau, "Plasmon enhanced energy transfer from a conjugated polymer to fluorescent core shell nanoparticles: a photophysical study", *J. Phys. Chem.*, vol. 115, pp. 2974-2981, 2011.

[64]   J. Asselin, M.L. Viger, and D. Boudreau, "Review article, metal-enhanced fluorescence and fret in multilayer core-shell nanoparticles, advances in chemistry", *Hindawi Publishing Corporation*, vol. 812313, pp. 1-16, 2014.

[65]   M.H. Chowdhury, S. Chakraborty, J.R. Lakowicz, and K. Ray, "Feasibility of using bimetallic plasmonic nanostructures to enhance the intrinsic emission of biomolecules", *J Phys Chem C Nanomater Interfaces*, vol. 115, no. 34, pp. 16879-16891, 2011.
[http://dx.doi.org/10.1021/jp205108s] [PMID: 21984954]

[66]   J. Zhang, Y. Fu, M.H. Chowdhury, and J.R. Lakowicz, "Metal-enhanced single-molecule fluorescence on silver particle monomer and dimer: coupling effect between metal particles", *Nano Lett.*, vol. 7, no. 7, pp. 2101-2107, 2007.
[http://dx.doi.org/10.1021/nl071084d] [PMID: 17580926]

[67]   Y. Liu, J. Bishop, L. Williams, S. Blair, and J. Herron, "Biosensing based upon molecular confinement in metallic nanocavity arrays", *Nanotechnology*, vol. 15, pp. 1368-1374, 2004.
[http://dx.doi.org/10.1088/0957-4484/15/9/043]

[68]   Y. Liu, and S. Blair, "Fluorescence enhancement from an array of subwavelength metal apertures", *Opt. Lett.*, vol. 28, no. 7, pp. 507-509, 2003.
[http://dx.doi.org/10.1364/OL.28.000507] [PMID: 12696598]

[69]   Q. Wei, G. Acuna, S. Kim, C. Vietz, D. Tseng, J. Chae, D. Shir, W. Luo, P. Tinnefeld, and A. Ozcan, *Plasmonics Enhanced Smartphone Fluorescence Microscopy*, vol. 7, no. 2124, 2017.
[http://dx.doi.org/10.1038/s41598-017-02395-8] [PMID: PMC5437072]

[70]   P. Song, J. H. Wang, M. Zhang, F. Yang, H. J. Lu, B. Kang, J. J. Xu, and H. Y. Chen, "Three level spaser for next generation luminescent nanoprobe", *Sci. Adv*, pp. 1-7, 2018.
[PMID: eaat0292]

[71]   G. Lerario, A. Fieramosca, F. Barachati, D. Ballarini, K. S. Daskalakis, L. Dominici, M. DeGiorgi, S. A. Maier, G. Gigli, S. Kéna-Cohen, and D. Sanvitto, "Room-temperature super fluidity in a polariton condensate",

[72]   D. M. Balazs, K. I. Bijlsma, H. H. Fang, D. N. Dirin, and M. Dobeli, " Stoichometric control of the density of states in PbS colloidal quanttum dot solids", *Sci. Adv,* vol. 3, pp. 1-7, 2017.
[http://dx.doi.org/] [PMID: eaao1558]

[73]   P. Lodahl, A. Floris Van Driel, I.S. Nikolaev, A. Irman, K. Overgaag, D. Vanmaekelbergh, and W.L. Vos, "Controlling the dynamics of spontaneous emission from quantum dots by photonic crystals", *Nature,* vol. 430, no. 7000, pp. 654-657, 2004.
[http://dx.doi.org/10.1038/nature02772] [PMID: 15295594]

[74]   D. Englund, D. Fattal, E. Waks, G. Solomon, B. Zhang, T. Nakaoka, Y. Arakawa, Y. Yamamoto, and J. Vuckovic, " Controlling the spontaneous emission rate of single Quantum Dots in a two dimension photonic crystals", *Physical Review Letters,* vol. 95, pp. 1-4, 2005.
[PMID: 013904]

[75]   D. Bera, L. Qian, T-K. Tseng, and P.H. Holloway, "Quantum dots and their multimodal applications: a review", *Materials (Basel),* vol. 3, pp. 2260-2345, 2010.
[http://dx.doi.org/10.3390/ma3042260]

[76]   A. Hatef, S. Fortin-Deschenes, E. Boulais, F. Lesage, and M. Meunier, "Photothermal response of hollow gold nanoshell to laser irradiation: continuous wave, short and ultrashort pulse", *Int. J. Heat Mass Transf.,* vol. 89, pp. 866-871, 2015.
[http://dx.doi.org/10.1016/j.ijheatmasstransfer.2015.05.071]

[77]   M. Reindl, D. Huber, C. Schimpf, S. F. Covre da Silve, M. B. Rota, H. Huang, V. Zwiller, K. D. Jons, A. Rastelli, and R. Trotta, "All photonic quantum teleportation using on demand solid state quantum emitters", *Sci. Adv,* vol. 4, pp. 1-7, 2018.
[PMID: eaau1255]

[78]   Y.H. Huo, A. Rastelli, and O.G. Schmidt, "Ultra-small excitonic fine structure splitting in highly symmetric quantum dots on GaAs (001) substrate", *Appl. Phys. Lett.,* vol. 102, no. 152105, pp. 1-4, 2013.
[http://dx.doi.org/10.1063/1.4802088]

[79]   M. Huo, J. Quin, J. Cheng, Z. Yan, Z. Yan, Z. Quin, X. Su, X. Jia, C. Xie, and K. Peng, "Deterministic quantum teleportation through fiber channels", *Sci. Adv,* vol. 4, pp. 1-7, 2018.
[PMID: eaas9401]

[80]   W.W. Chow, "Quantum-optical influences in optoelectronics—An introduction", *Appl. Phys. Rev.,* vol. 5, no. 041302, pp. 1-21, 2018.

[81]   T. Nitsche, S. Barkhofen, R. Kruse, L. Sansoni, M. Stefanak, A. Gabris, V. Potocek, T. Kiss, I. Jex, and C. Silberhorn, *Sci. Adv,* vol. 4, pp. 1-8, 2018.
[PMID: eaar6444]

[82]   X. Shi, W. You, Y. Zhang, Z. Tao, P. M. Oppeneer, X. Wu, R. Thomale, K. Rossnagel, M. Bauer, H. Kapteyn, and M. Murnane, "Ultrafast electron calorimetry uncovers a new long lived metastable state in 1T-TaSe2 mediated by mode selective electron phonon coupling", *Sci. Adv,* vol. 5, no. , pp. 1-7, 2019.
[http://dx.doi.org/] [PMID: eaav4449]

[83]   C. Jia, M. Famili, M. Carlotti, Y. Liu, P. Wang, L. M. Grace, Z. Feng, Y. Wang, Z. Zhao, M. Ding, X. Xu, C. Wang, S. J. Lee, Y. Huang, R. C. Chiechi, C. J. Lambert, and X. Duang, "Quantum interference mediated vertical molecular tunneling transistors", *Sci. Adv,* vol. 4, pp. 1-8, 2018.
[PMID: eaat8237]

CHAPTER 5

Developments in Nanophotonics

Abstract: In this chapter it is shown and discussed how luminescent emission for low molecular concentrations and targeted DNA detection, detection of individual biostructure and nanolaser fabrication for biophotonics, genomics, nanomedicine and nanotechnological applications can be transduced and improved on the basis of major research studies on the design of several nanoarchitectures, nano-patterned surfaces and their interaction with different light excitations.

Keywords: Biophotonics, DNA detection, Enhanced luminescent core-shell nanoparticles, Enhanced luminescent supramolecular nanoparticles, Genomics, Molecular detection, Nanophotonics, Ultraluminescent bio labelling, Ultraluminescent nanoarchitectures.

1. DEVELOPMENTS IN NANOPHOTONICS

The control of the nanoscale and the study of light interaction with the nanomaterials designed should aim at targeted applications, such as different types of nanoarchitectures. In this section, we attempt to describe major developments, including the design of functional nanoplatforms based on different criteria according to specific uses. In addition, the design, synthesis and optimization and iteration of whole processes are shown.

2. ULTRALUMINESCENT FUNCTIONAL NANOMATERIALS

Functional nanomaterials could be incorporated in colloidal dispersion systems, modified surfaces as well as in-flow methodologies and studied by different optical approaches depending on the physical and chemical signals tracked. In particular, the use of luminescent probes or labellers has allowed high sensitivity due to the intrinsic characteristics of this technique. However, new advanced approaches are still in progress in order to overcome optical limitations and improve signal and functionalities.

Consequently, within this challenging field, modified plasmonic surfaces were studied in the UV region for enhanced fluorescence of proteins and label-free bioassays using aluminum nanostructures [1] Immobilized protein molecules on the surface of a nanostructured aluminum film resulted in a significant improvement of fluorescence intensity (up to 14-fold) and decrease in a lifetime (up to 6-fold) compared to quartz substrates.

In colloidal dispersion, stable and well dispersed Indium@silica core-shell Nanoparticles were accurately designed as plasmonic enhancers of molecular luminescence in the UV region [2]. Fluorescence measurements for In@SiO2@SiO2Carbostyril 124 and In@SiO2@SiO2-tryptophan immobilized on nanocomposites with 5 and 12 nm thick silica spacer shells, respectively, caused fluorescence enhancement of 5 and 7, respectively, in comparison to core-less nanoarchitectures. Thus, enhancement factors were improved, ranging from 1.3 to 3 in the N-acetyl tryptophan amide derivative using vapour-deposited indium nanoscopy. Films as reported previously [3].

Moreover, the generation of high luminescent emission from reduced sizes is of high interest within the nanoscalefor multimodal nanoimaging, bioimaging and nanomedicine. In this way, biocompatible gold core-shell nanoparticles were designed by the incorporation of a laser dye sensitizer such as Rhodamine B (RhB) on silanized spacers (Au@SiO$_2$-RhB) [4]. These nanoparticles showed ultraluminescent properties with enhancements in colloidal dispersion, from single nanoparticle analysis by laser fluorescence microscopy based on the Metal Enhanced Fluorescence (MEF) effect. These Au@SiO$_2$-RhB nanoparticles were used as ultraluminescent biolabellers for individual bacterial detection based on metal-enhanced fluorescence nanoimaging [4]. These new nanomaterials are still being developed and are a part of many plasmonic nanoarchitectures linked to other research fields such as photonic nanomaterials applied to the transference and storage of high energy in the near field for far field applications [5].

Less time-consuming methodologies with higher sensitivity include free PCR analysis and single molecule detection (**SMD**). In this field, we could refer to plasmon-controlled fluorescence and single DNA strand sequencing [6] based on modified plasmonic aluminium nanostructured surfaces, *in vivo* single molecule imaging of bacterial DNA replication and transcription and repair [7] by laser fluorescence microscopy.

Another type of nanomaterials with varied composition depending on requirements comprises photonic crystal protein hydrogel sensor for Candida albicans [8]], tunable fluorescence of a semiconducting polythiophene located on DNA origami [9] and plasmonic origamies [10] with potential applications in enhanced luminescent surfaces and incorporation into microdevices.

As shown, the importance of the control of light lies in the fact that there could be other strategies, approaches and designs for improved performance, such as the 2014 Nobel prize-awarded development, in chemistry, of super-resolved fluorescence microscopy, shared by USA and Germany [11], and the 2018 Nobel Prize-awarded tools made of light, in physics, shared by USA, France and Canada [12]. In all the cases illustrated, based on the development of nanomaterial, control was achieved on photon emission depending on the interval of emission wavelengths or targeted reporter.

3. ENHANCED ULTRALUMINESCENT MULTILAYERED NANOPLATFORMS

For the design of ultraluminescent functional nanomaterials applied to signal transductions, multiple physical phenomena could be coupled, as it was previously discussed with core-shell nanoparticles. In a similar manner, the design of optical transparent materials coupled to optical resonators, such as Resonant plasmonic cores applied to **MEF**. In this way, multilayered core-shell nanoparticles were developed from a strong plasmonic silver core covered with a modified and optimized first silica spacer shell for **MEF** of a fluorescent energy acceptor, incorporating a second silica spacer shell as **fluorescence Energy** donor [13]. The spectroscopical properties of the donor/acceptor pairs added were well overlapped to exploit **FRET** enhancement.

Hence, the excitation at 488 nm Laser excitation, the fluorescent polymer energy donor was first coupled by enhanced **FRET** from the interaction of the fluorescent energy donor-plasmonic core and then by donor/acceptor **FRET-MEF**. The multilayer core-shell nanoparticles showed diminished photobleaching properties and higher intense emission as compared with absence of the fluorescent energy donor layer. Their markedly improved luminosity made them promising optical probes for a variety of applications such as cell imaging and biosensing.

Another multi-layered core-shell nanoarchitecture was reported from a gold core surrounded with CdSe quantum dot donors and S101 dyes as acceptors to exploit **FRET** phenomenon [14]. The multilayer configuration exhibited synergistic effects of surface plasmon energy transfer from the metal to the CdSe and plasmon-enhanced **FRET** from the quantum dots to the dye. With precise control over the distance between the components in the nanostructure, significant improvement in the emission of CdSe was achieved by combined resonance energy transfer and near-field enhancement by the metal, as well as subsequent improvement in the emission of dye induced by the enhanced emission of CdSe. In genomics, such as Free PCR assays, a lab-on particle nanostructure for label-free biosensing was designed from chemical and biochemically modified multilayer fluorescent nanocomposites and a cationic polymeric transducer [15] for DNA genotyping applications. This nanoarchitecture was based on a modified silver core-shell nanoparticle with different functionalized layers for enhanced **FRET** signal transduction and detection. The first layered core-shell nanoarchitecture used a **MEF** nanoplatform for targeted DNA strand grafting accurately separated by a second silica spacer shell from the acceptor layer for optimal **FRET**.

The fluorescent energy reporter was an intercalated fluorescent poly-thiophene within the grafted single DNA strands. These fluorescent polymer-DNA dimmers showed lower quantum yields in the absence of the complementary DNA strand. After interaction with the targeted DNA strand, an increased quantum yield was determined [16]. Hence, in the presence of the complementary targeted DNA strand, enhanced emissions were recorded *via* a supramolecular enhanced structural arrangement, through **FRET**-**MEF** coupling. Note that the nanoarchitectures referring above to genotyping assays were developed within an in-flow cytometry coupled to an enhanced optical approach with camera for detection and analysis of individual nanoparticles [15]. Therefore, enhanced approaches are highly required in order to track interactions within confined spaces.

In this field, we should highlight the concept of miniaturization as well as the incorporation of proof of concepts and modified and standard methodologies within 90 microdevices. A recent report showed portable infrared isothermal PCR platform for strand detection of multiple sexually transmitted diseases [17]. This platform consisted of a multi-chamber microfluidic chip for simultaneous amplification and testing detection. This microfluidic chip integrated RNA extraction, micro-pump and multi- target detection in the same chip. By application of IR light-emitting diode (LED) as a heat source, this platform could fulfil isothermal amplification within 70 minutes. These enhancements and energy transduction across the nanomaterials could also be applied to other applications in confined spaces, such as nanofluidic and microfluidic systems, silica waveguides and modified silica wave guides with incorporation of other components, as well as in other lab-on chip configurations and nanophotonic arrays that will be discussed in the next sections.

In this way the potential of the design of microdevices was shown to be coupled to well-known modified biochemical procedures and improved routine analysis. Thus, this concept could be extended to individual nanophotonic platforms and analysis for a large number of applications.

3.1. Nanolasers and Nanoantennas

The control of size and shape of nanomaterials by wet-chemical methods over surfaces or in colloidal dispersion and nanolithography techniques has allowed the development of nanoarchitectures with different material properties. In particular, nanorods showed non-homogeneous plasmonic and emission properties according to the nanomaterial and media used. Resonance wavelength depended on the orientation of the electric field relative to the particle, and thus, oscillations either along (longitudinal) or across (transversal) the rod were determined [17].

Because of the dimensionality of anisotropic shapes, the frequencies associated with the various resonance modes can differ considerably, and consequently, the optical properties can be largely affected. These resonances could be theorically calculated and modeled using the equations derived by Mie for the resolution of Maxwell equations for the absorption and scattering of electromagnetic radiation by small spheres [18] and their modifications by Gans for ellipsoids [19]. Many studies reported strong plasmonic intensities within the IR region along the rods later applied to the design of new nanomaterials, as in photonic surfaces.

The development of modified surfaces with highly organized and nano-patterned gold nanorods led to new hyperbolic metamaterial properties with strong lasing phenomenon, producing 35% higher emissions than those of elliptical 92 arrays [20] (Fig. **1**). Hence, hyperbolic metamaterials can serve as a convenient platform and source of coherent photon generation/development in a broad wavelength range.

This effect was observed on grated films with noble nanorods that produced a superluminality phenomenon at a femtosecond laser pulse propagation through this medium [21]. It was demonstrated that the fast light propagation occurred within wave packet carriers and resonance frequencies from inter-nanoparticle interactions as a chirped phenomenon.

Other common nanomaterials involve geometries as nano-wires, rods and other polygonal geometries based on cooper, zinc, aluminium, silver nanostructures and semiconductor materials, with varied conductive and radiative properties. Thus, nanolaser properties from ZnO nanorods based on natural resonance cavities [22] obtained on patterned gold layers deposited on GaN/Al_2O_3 substrates were evaluated by applying different irradiancy power-generated strong photo-emitting surfaces. Moreover, semiconductor materials such as InGaAsP iron-nail-shaped rod-type structures were embedded in PDMS to obtain flexible high-resolution strain-gauge nanolasers.

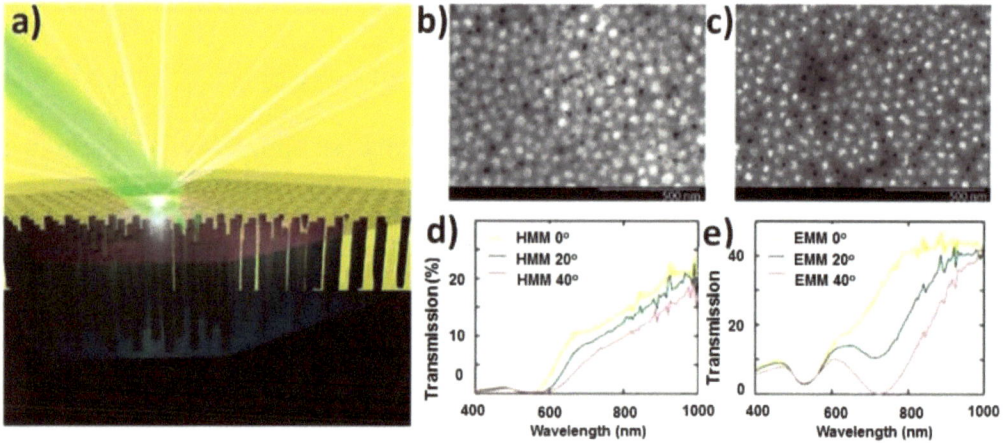

Fig. (1). a) Scheme of lasing action from nanorod-based metamaterials. **b, c)** Top-view SEM images of hyperbolic metamaterial (HMM) and elliptic metamaterial (EMM), with metal fill ratios of 35% and 14%, respectively. **d, e)** Transmission spectra of HMM and EMM illuminated with TM-polarized light at 0°, 20°, and 40° incidence [21].

In addition, from studies based on tuning of single nanorod mode lasing, ultralow threshold properties were recorded for multi-wavelength plasmonics [23]. These nanolasers were based on a single metal-oxide-semiconductor nanostructure platform comprising InGaN/GaN semiconductor nanorods supported on an Al_2O_3-capped epitaxial Ag film. All-color lasing in subdiffraction plasmonic resonators was achieved *via* a novel mechanism based on weak size dependence inherent in spasers.

Another nanotechnological approach, based on a nano-patterning control, centers on the concept of nanoantennas from inter-nanoparticle interaction, for example, dimeric nanorods as strong antenna enhanced fluorescence of single light harvesters [24]. Thus, signals could be transduced and enhanced in terms of the strategy used or the targeted application of the nanomaterial.

These phenomena from the near field related to shorter lengths between nanostructures are very close to the quantum scale and regime. For these reasons studies into the frontiers of quantics and plasmonics are still being developed. A recently published study indicated collective modes of quantum fluids related to new plasmons and emerging quantum states, in the fractional quantum Hall regime named as intra-Landau-level plasmons, measured by resonant inelastic light scattering [25]. From these new nanomaterials, coupled phenomena and advanced nano- and microdevices could be designed, studied and developed. This field is, therefore, opening up to novel 94 possibilities. Other non-classical materials involve quantum materials such as disks and nanowires with nanoscale cathode luminescence properties [26], which could be incorporated into microdevices as emitting ring quantum cascade lasers for, say, chemical sensing [27].

3.2. Supramolecular Nanoparticles

Supramolecular chemistry, defined as the chemistry of the non-covalent interactions generated varied molecular host-guest complementarities applied to the design of functional molecular devices and synthesis of molecular machines. In relation to this, a Nobel prize in Chemistry was awarded to France in 1987 [28] and in 2016 to France, Netherlands and United Kingdom [29], respectively. These sub-nanometer supramolecular architectures beyond molecular sizes and below 1.0 nm have led to studies of molecular interactions based on different non-covalent host-guest complexes.

The most well-known supramolecular systems such as macrocycles with well-defined cavities comprise calixarenes [30] (**CA**), cucurbiturils [30] (**CB**) and cyclodextrins [30] (**CD**). All these receptors have a nanocavity with different organic groups that can interact with the guest included. For instance, cyclodextrins (**CDs**) are cyclic oligosaccharides consisting of six (**αCD**), seven (**ßCD**) or eight (**γCD**) units of [31]. α–D-glucose linked by α- (1,4) bonds. These macrocycles have a nanocavity (internal diameter of 0.7 nm for **ßCD**) which allows them to act as hosts to form inclusion complexes with guest molecules in the solid state or in solution. **CDs** are interesting microvessels capable of embedding appropriately sized molecules; the resulting supramolecules can serve as excellent miniature models for enzyme-substratecomplexes. These sub-nanometer chemical structures synthesized from molecules have allowed the development of different nanomaterials and applications [30], such as thesmart multifunctional nanoparticles for sensors and drug delivery systems [31]. Here, we should highlight their implication in complex formation with different organic and inorganic fluorescent reporter dyes as well as their contribution as non-covalent linkers, being, hence, constitutive parts of nanoparticles. From these interactions and bottom-up approaches, many developments within nanophotonics and potential applications with the control of light were reported. A case in point constitutes light-driven artificial molecular machines [32] (Fig. **2**) which, by a control of reversible molecular motions in artificial molecular machines, enable switch on/off enhanced fluorescence control and molecular release using simple chemistry reactions based on hybrid gold supramolecular nanoparticles [32].

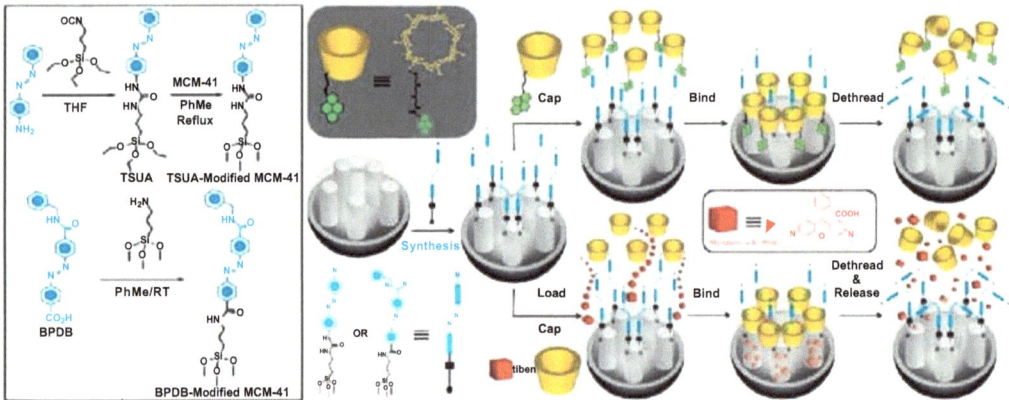

Fig. (2). Artificial molecular machines work as nanovalves for drug delivery. Py-βCD or β-CD threads onto the trans-AB stalks to seal the nanopores βCyclodextrin: βCD). Upon irradiation (351 nm), isomerization of trans-to-cis AB units leads to dissociation of Py-β-CD or β-CD rings from stalks, thus the gates opening to the nanopores and releasing the cargo. Reprinted with permission from T. J. Huang *et al.* Copyright 2010 Journal of Nanophotonics, SPIE [32].

It should be noted that many supramolecular complexes could increase the fluorescence emissions of the guest incorporated, as in indoles [33], carbamate [34] and anthracene derivatives [35], in addition to other organic molecules. However, fluorescence quenching could also be reported, for example, in the presence of Rhodamine-βCD complexes [36]. In this sense, depending on needs and appropriate development and tuning of the different parts of nanoparticles, these properties could be even improved and used of targeted applications, such as metal enhanced fluorescence (**MEF**) emission and quenching protection effect of Rhodamine-βCD complexes based on βCD grafted gold nanophotonic platforms [37].

These nanoplatforms showed varied inter-nanoparticle interactions in view of the molecular spacers used and the polarity of the media that generated/formed tuneable plasmonic properties, from individual plasmonic resonance to enhanced plasmonics for **MEF** detection [38]. At this point it should be noted that, from molecular recognition at a defined distance from the gold nanoplatform, the well-known quenching effect of the complexed Rhodamine B used as molecular reporter with the macrocyclic receptor was overcome.

Other approaches combining different macrocycles and complexes can be included in the design of mechanized mesoporous silica nanoparticles. The proof of the principle level was demonstrated on cyclodextrins and cucurbiturils, leading to cargo release from the inside of nanoparticles [39], potentially applied to light tracked drug delivery. Nanoplatforms for fluorescent nanoimaging and drug delivery applications can also be mentioned, as in β-Cyclodextrin-bearing gold glyconanoparticles for the development of site-specific drug delivery systems [40] and protein-sized bright fluorogenic nanoparticles based on crosslinked calixarene micelles with Cyanine Corona [41].

In addition, another targeted light tracking could be designed based on fluorescent nanoparticles. Most of the current bacterial detection methods are time-consuming and laborious and can detect only one bacterial pathogen at a time. Accordingly, by the appropriate tuning of fluorescent nanoparticles, multiplexed bacteria were monitored.

These nanoparticles consisted of multicolored **FRET** (fluorescence resonance energy transfer) silica nanoparticles, modified with monoclonal specific antibodies for pathogenic bacteria species such as *Escherichia coli*, *Salmonella typhimurium* and *Staphylococcus aureus*. These nanoparticles were rapid, sensitive and selective for pathogenic bacteria detection, which is particularly important for proper containment, diagnosis and treatment of diseases like food borne illness, sepsis and bioterrorism.

Another nanoarchitecture combining plasmonic, supramolecular and polymeric properties can be mentioned: optical detection of antibody using silica-silver core-shell nanoparticles [43]. These nanoparticles were formed by a silica core decorated with silver nanoparticles, conjugated with antibodies. The silver-grafted nanoparticles showed strong surface plasmon resonance peaks at 453 nm, shifted in the presence of anti-antibody interactions. In this case, the silica nanoparticles were solid supports of plasmonics properties and supramolecular modifications allowed the development of the hybrid silica supramolecular nanoparticles. Finally, we should report the development of new supramolecular polymers for potential applications in nanophotonics as well [44].

3.3. From Single Nanoparticle Spectroscopy to Nanoarray Analysis

The development of nanoparticles in colloidal dispersion by wet-chemistry methods, their deposition over modified surfaces or by nanolithography techniques has allowed obtaining varied nanoparticle dispersibility with controlled assembly and nanopatterning, respectively, as discussed in the preceding sections. These systems based on different optical detection techniques such as fluorescence microscopy [45], dark-field microscopy [46], near-field microscopy [47] and other advanced optical approaches, such as optical tweezers [48], have allowed spectroscopical detection and characterization from individual nanoplatforms to photonic surface analysis from nanoarrays.

In order to achieve these types of analysis, other techniques and their limitations should be described so as to propose new nanoarchitectures and optical strategies and approaches. Thus, even if this broadens the scope of the section, the basis of the optical setups of microscopy and their limitations need to be discussed.

In this manner, in order to obtain detailed images and high resolution of nanoimages applied to biolabelling for biodetection and bioimaging generation, the resolution limit of optical microscopes should be improved [49]. The possible minimum distance (d) between two structural elements that could be conceived such as two objects instead of one is given by $d = \lambda / (2NA)$, where λ is the wavelength of light and NA is the numerical aperture of the objective lens. This parameter, in optimal conditions with white light, the resolution of optical microscopes can reach 250 nm. For this reason, for microstructure detection, only optical microscopes are required.

Yet, if detection of individual biological microstructures with improved detail from image analysis is needed, developments in this way are called for enhanced resolution, new optical approaches are being developed, applying fluorescence microscopy, including selective imaging of surface fluorescence with very high aperture microscope objectives [50] and *in vivo* fluorescence imaging with high-resolution microlenses [51].

Moreover, the combination of optics and plasmonics gives the possibility of addressing problems related to signal dispersion, transduction and final resolution, as in surface plasmon resonance imaging using a high numerical aperture microscope objective [52]. Consequently, developments in the labelling of biological surfaces are desired/required by using the most sophisticated commercial microscopes. Additionally, these approaches can be easily applied to biodetection with commercial in-flow instruments using fluorescence detection and imaging. They can also be included in new optical arrays to further enhance the resolution of the images obtained from the biological event detection. The challenge posed for nanoimaging resolution by fluorescence is to tune the appropriate ratio of nanodimension and luminescence intensity to allow surface labelling and reduce fluorescence intensity overlapping between different nanoparticles when they are so close; however they should be intense enough for individual nanoparticle and bacteria labelled tracking with a small number of nanoparticles per ml. One of the principal parameters to take into account is lateral resolution [53], in which the point separation (r) in the image plane is the distance between the central maximum and the first minimum intensity from an individual nanoparticle imaging: $r_{lateral} = 1.22 \times \lambda/(2 \times NA) = 0.6 \times \lambda/NA$, where λ is the emitted light wavelength and NA is the numerical aperture of the objective.

An improved detail from image analysis is particularly important for many reasons, mainly for plasma membrane topography and interpretation of single particle tracking over the surface [54], based on single particle tracking (SPT) by light microscopy on live cells and electron microscopy, where the importance of membrane constitution and topography [55] in the folding process was demonstrated.

In view of this, if possible, detection of biological microstructure or nanostructure and collection of information thoroughly detailed from image analysis should be sought. In this sense, it will be easier to arrive at fast and no time-consuming diagnostics. Another example of the importance of biostructure detection for a specific and immediately consecutive analysis was developed by Weissleder *et al.* (2013), applied to the detection and genotyping of new bacteria. From this viewpoint, new nanosensors integrated in high-impact microdevice developments have been fostered for social needs. This is the case of microdevices for integration of bacterial detection, such as magneto-DNA nanoparticle system for rapid detection and phenotyping of bacteria by PCR [56].

Within this field, the design of multifunctional nanoparticles as important toolkits for fluorescent cell and bacteria labelling as well for molecular biodetection is of widespread and increasing interest in technological applications coupled to new optical approaches, and their incorporation into microdevices. To illustrate this, we can bring up the use of gold/thiol functionalized within conducting and stretchable nanometer-thin polydimethylsiloxane films [57] and the design of multi-analyte resonant photonic platform for label-free biosensing [58]. Here, the basis and concepts of micro-chip designs and modifications could be obtained from specific procedures and manipulations.

CONCLUDING REMARKS

By the control of size and shape of nanomaterials, along with the right chemical modifications, it was possible to tune enhanced emissions from smart responsive interactions. In this way, low molecular detection was recorded at single molecular detection **(SMD)** levels and ultraluminescent surfaces were developed for nanophotonics, biophotonics and nanotechnological applications.

REFERENCES

[1]   K. Ray, H. Szmacinski, and J.R. Lakowicz, "Enhanced fluorescence of proteins and label-free bioassays using aluminum nanostructures", *Anal. Chem,* vol. 81, no. 15, pp. 6049-6054, 2009. [http://dx.doi.org/10.1021/ac900263k] [PMID: 19594133]

[2]   F. Magnan, J. Gagnon, F-G. Fontaine, and D. Boudreau, "Indium@silica core-shell nanoparticles as plasmonic enhancers of molecular luminescence in the UV region", *Chem. Commun. (Camb.),* vol. 49, no. 81, pp. 9299-9301, 2013. [http://dx.doi.org/10.1039/c3cc45276j] [PMID: 23999800]

[3]   A.I. Dragan, and C.D. Geddes, "Indium nanodeposits: A substrate for metal enhanced fluorescence in the ultraviolet spectral region", *J. Appl. Phys.,* vol. 108, no. 094701, pp. 1-7, 2010.
[http://dx.doi.org/10.1063/1.3503439]

[4]   D. Gontero, A. V. Veglia, D. Boudreau, and A. G. Bracamonte, "Ultraluminescent gold Core-shell nanoparticles applied to individual bacterial detection based on Metal-Enhanced Fluorescence Nanoimaging", *J. of Nanophotonics. Special issue Nanoplasmonics for Biosensing, Enhanced Light-Matter Interaction, and Spectral Engineering,* vol. 12,1, no. 012505, pp. 1-12, 2018.

[5]   A.G. Bracamonte, "Design of new Photonic Nanomaterials applied to the transference and storage of high Energy in the near and far field", *Bitácora digital Journal. Energy,* vol. 4, 8° EdFaculty of Chem. Sc. (UNC), pp. 1-18, 2017.

[6]   N. Akbay, K. Ray, M.H. Chowdhury, and J.R. Lakowicz, "Plasmon-controlled fluorescence and single DNA strand sequenching", *Proc SPIE Int Soc Opt Eng,* vol. 8234, no. 82340M, p. 82340M, 2012.
[http://dx.doi.org/10.1117/12.916177] [PMID: 24027614]

[7]   M. Stracy, S. Uphoff, F. Garza de Leon, and A.N. Kapanidis, "*In vivo* single-molecule imaging of bacterial DNA replication, transcription, and repair", *FEBS Lett.,* vol. 588, no. 19, pp. 3585-3594, 2014.
[http://dx.doi.org/10.1016/j.febslet.2014.05.026] [PMID: 24859634]

[8]   Z. Cai, D.H. Kwak, D. Punihaole, Z. Hong, S.S. Velankar, X. Liu, and S.A. Asher, "A photonic crystal protein hydrogel sensor for candida albicans", *Angew. Chem. Int. Ed. Engl.,* vol. 54, no. 44, pp. 13036-13040, 2015.
[http://dx.doi.org/10.1002/anie.201506205] [PMID: 26480336]

[9]   J. Zessin, F. Fischer, A. Heerwig, A. Kick, S. Boye, M. Stamm, A. Kiriy, and M. Mertig, "Tunable fluorescence of a semiconducting polythiophene positioned on DNA origami", *Nano Lett.,* vol. 17, no. 8, pp. 5163-5170, 2017.
[http://dx.doi.org/10.1021/acs.nanolett.7b02623] [PMID: 28745060]

[10]   P. Wang, S. Gaitanaros, S. Lee, M. Bathe, W.M. Shih, and Y. Ke, "Programming self-assembly of DNA origami honeycomb two-dimensional lattices and plasmonic metamaterials", *J. Am. Chem. Soc.,* vol. 138, no. 24, pp. 7733-7740, 2016.
[http://dx.doi.org/10.1021/jacs.6b03966] [PMID: 27224641]

[11]   E. Betzig, S.W. Hell, and W.E. Moerner, "The nobel prize in chemistry 2014, for the development of super-resolved fluorescence microscopy", *Press Release of The Royal Swedish Academy of Sciences,* 2014.

[12]   A. Ashkin, G. Mourou, and D. Strickland, "The Nobel Prize in Physics 2018, tools made of light: for their method of generating high-intensity, ultra-short optical pulses", *Press Release of The Royal Swedish Academy of Sciences,* 2018.

[13]   M. Lessard-Viger, M. Rioux, L. Rainville, and D. Boudreau, "FRET enhancement in multilayer core-shell nanoparticles", *Nano Lett.,* vol. 9, no. 8, pp. 3066-3071, 2009.
[http://dx.doi.org/10.1021/nl901553u] [PMID: 19603786]

[14]   S. T. Kochuveedu1,T. Son,Y. Lee,M. Lee, Dong, "Revolutionizing the fret-based light emission in core-shell nanostructures via comprehensive activity of surface plasmons", *Sci. Rep.,* vol. 4, no. 4735, pp. 1-8, 2014.

[15]   D. Brouard, M.L. Viger, A.G. Bracamonte, and D. Boudreau, "Label-free biosensing based on multilayer fluorescent nanocomposites and a cationic polymeric transducer", *ACS Nano,* vol. 5, no. 3, pp. 1888-1896, 2011.
[http://dx.doi.org/10.1021/nn102776m] [PMID: 21344882]

[16]   M.B. Abérem, A. Najari, H-A. Ho, J-F. Gravel, P. Nobert, D. Boudreau, and M. Leclerc, "Protein detecting arrays based on cationic polythiophene– DNA-aptamer complexes", *Adv. Mater.,* vol. 18, pp. 2703-2707, 2006.

[http://dx.doi.org/10.1002/adma.200601651]

[17]   J. Perez-Juste, I. Pastoriza-Santos, L.M. Liz-Marzan, and P. Mulvaney, "Gold nanorods: synthesis, characterization and applications", *Coord. Chem. Rev.,* vol. 249, pp. 1870-1901, 2005.
[http://dx.doi.org/10.1016/j.ccr.2005.01.030]

[18]   G. Mie, "Beiträge zur Optik trüber Medien, speziell kolloidaler Metallösungen", *Ann. Phys.,* vol. 25, p. 377, 1908.
[http://dx.doi.org/10.1002/andp.19083300302]

[19]   R. Gans, "Über die Form ultramikroskopischer Goldteilchen", *Ann. Phys.,* vol. 37, p. 881, 1912.
[http://dx.doi.org/10.1002/andp.19123420503]

[20]   R. Chandrasekar, Z. Wang, X. Meng, S.I. Azzam, M.Y. Shalaginov, A. Lagutchev, Y.L. Kim, A. Wei, A.V. Kildishev, A. Boltasseva, and V.M. Shalaev, "Lasing action with gold nanorod hyperbolic metamaterials", *ACS Photonics,* vol. 4, pp. 674-680, 2017.
[http://dx.doi.org/10.1021/acsphotonics.7b00010]

[21]   V. A. Trofimov, and T. M. Lysak, "Superluminality phenomenon at a femtosecond laser pulse propagation in a medium containing nanorods", *J. Nanophoton,* vol. 11, 2, no. 026003, pp. 1-25, 2017.

[22]   G. Visimberga, E.E. Yakimov, A.N. Redkin, A.N. Gruzintsev, V.T. Volkov, S. Romanov, and G.A. Emelchenko, "Nanolasers from ZnO nanorods as natural resonance cavities", *Phys. Status Solidi., C Curr. Top. Solid State Phys.,* vol. 7, no. 6, pp. 1668-1671, 2010.
[http://dx.doi.org/10.1002/pssc.200983156]

[23]   Y.J. Lu, C.Y. Wang, J. Kim, H.Y. Chen, M.Y. Lu, Y.C. Chen, W.H. Chang, L.J. Chen, M.I. Stockman, C.K. Shih, S. Gwo, and Lu Y.-Jung, "All-color plasmonic nanolasers with ultralow thresholds: autotuning mechanism for single-mode lasing", *Nano Lett.,* vol. 14, no. 8, pp. 4381-4388, 2014.
[http://dx.doi.org/10.1021/nl501273u] [PMID: 25029207]

[24]   E. Wientjes, J. Renger, A.G. Curto, R. Cogdell, and N.F. van Hulst, "Strong antenna-enhanced fluorescence of a single light-harvesting complex shows photon antibunching", *Nat. Commun.,* vol. 5, no. 4236, p. 4236, 2014.
[http://dx.doi.org/10.1038/ncomms5236] [PMID: 24953833]

[25]   L. Du, U. Wurstbauer, K. W. West, L. N. Pfeiffer, S. Fallahi, G. C. Gardiner, M. J. Manfra, and A. Pinczuk, "Observation of new plasmons in the fractional quantum Hall effect: Interplay of topological and nematic orders", *Adv,* vol. 5, no. eaav340, pp. 1-6, 2019.

[26]   Stowe Bilal A. Prabaswara D. J. , Ng J. Tien Khee, Anjum D. H., Zhao P. Longo C., Elafandy R. T., Ahmed X. Li, Munir Y. A., El-Desouki M., and Ooi B. S., "Spatially resolved investigation of competing nanocluster emission in quantum-disks-in-nanowires structure characterized by nanoscale cathodoluminescence", *J. Nanophoton,* vol. 11,2, no. 026015, pp. 1-13, 2017.

[27]   R. Szedlak, J. Hayden, P. Martín-Mateos, M. Holzbauer, A. Harrer, B. Schwarz, B. Hinkov, D. MacFarland, T. Zederbauer, H. Detz, A. Maxwell Andrews, W. Schrenk, P. Acedo, B. Lendl, and G. Strasser, "Surface emitting ring quantum cascade lasers for chemical sensing", *Opt. Eng,* vol. 57,1, no. 011005, pp. 1-5, 2017.

[28]   J. Lehn M., "Supramolecular Chemistry—Scope and Perspectives Molecules, Supermolecules, and Molecular Devices (Nobel Lecture)", *Angew. Chem. Int. Ed. Engl,* vol. 2, no. 71, pp. 89-112, 1988.

[29]   J-P. Sauvage, J.F. Stoddart, and B.L. Feringa, "The Nobel Prize in Chemistry 2016, for the design and synthesis of molecular machines", *Press Release by The Royal Swedish Academy of Sciences,* 2016.

[30]   J. W. Steed, and A.Gale Philip, "Supramolecular chemistry: from molecules to nanomaterials",

[31]   D. Gontero, M. Lessard-Viger, D. Brouard, A.G. Bracamonte, D. Boudreau, and A.V. Veglia, "Smart multifunctional nanoparticles design as sensors and drug delivery systems based on supramolecular chemistry", *Microchem. J.,* vol. 130, pp. 316-328, 2017.
[http://dx.doi.org/10.1016/j.microc.2016.10.007]

[32] Y. Bing, Z. Qingzhen, H. Ying-Wei, and B. Yang, Kiraly, I-K. Chiang, T. J. Huang, "Light-driven artificial molecular machines", *J. Nanophotonics*, vol. 4, no. 042501, pp. 1-27, 2010.

[33] A.G. Bracamonte, and A.V. Veglia, "Spectrofluorimetric determination of serotonin and 5-hydroxyindoleacetic acid in urine with different cyclodextrin media", *Talanta*, vol. 83, no. 3, pp. 1006-1013, 2011.
[http://dx.doi.org/10.1016/j.talanta.2010.11.013] [PMID: 21147351]

[34] N. L. Pacioni, and A. V. Veglia, "Determination of poorly fluorescent carbamate pesticides in water, bendiocarb and promecarb, using cyclodextrin nanocavities and related media, Analytica Chimica Acta",

[35] V.N. Sueldo Occello, and A.V. Veglia, "Cucurbit[6]uril nanocavity as an enhanced spectrofluorimetric method for the determination of pyrene", *Anal. Chim. Acta*, vol. 689, no. 1, pp. 97-102, 2011.
[http://dx.doi.org/10.1016/j.aca.2011.01.027] [PMID: 21338763]

[36] I. R. Politzer, K. T. Crago, T. Hampton, J. Joseph, J. H. Boyer, and M. Shah, "Effect of β-cyclodextrin on the fluorescence, absorption and lasing of rhodamine 6G, rhodamine B and fluorescein disodium salt in aqueous solutions", *Chemical Physics Letters*, vol. 159, no. 7, pp. 258-262, 1989. 2-3

[37] A.V. Veglia, and A. G. Bracamonte, "Metal enhanced fluorescence emission and quenching protection effect with a host-guest Nanophotonic-supramolecular structure", *Journal of Nanophotonics, Special Section on Nanoscience and Biomaterials in Photonics*, vol. 12,3, no. 033004, pp. 1-22, 2018.

[38] A.V. Veglia, and A.G. Bracamonte, "β-Cyclodextrin grafted gold nanoparticles with short molecular spacers applied for nanosensors based on plasmonic effects", *Microchem. J.*, vol. 148, pp. 277-284, 2019.
[http://dx.doi.org/10.1016/j.microc.2019.04.066]

[39] M.W. Ambrogio, T.A. Pecorelli, K. Patel, N.M. Khashab, A. Trabolsi, H.A. Khatib, Y.Y. Botros, J.I. Zink, and J.F. Stoddart, "Snap-top nanocarriers", *Org. Lett.*, vol. 12, no. 15, pp. 3304-3307, 2010.
[http://dx.doi.org/10.1021/ol101286a] [PMID: 20608669]

[40] A. Aykaç, M.C. Martos-Maldonado, J.M. Casas-Solvas, I. Quesada-Soriano, F. García-Maroto, L. García-Fuentes, and A. Vargas-Berenguel, "β-Cyclodextrin-bearing gold glyconanoparticles for the development of site specific drug delivery systems", *Langmuir*, vol. 30, no. 1, pp. 234-242, 2014.
[http://dx.doi.org/10.1021/la403454p] [PMID: 24313322]

[41] I. Shulov, R.V. Rodik, Y. Arntz, A. Reisch, V.I. Kalchenko, and A.S. Klymchenko, "Protein-sized bright fluorogenic nanoparticles based on cross-linked calixarene micelles with cyanine corona", *Angew. Chem. Int. Ed. Engl.*, vol. 55, no. 51, pp. 15884-15888, 2016.
[http://dx.doi.org/10.1002/anie.201609138] [PMID: 27862803]

[42] L. Wang, W. Zhao, M.B. O'Donoghue, and W. Tan, "Fluorescent nanoparticles for multiplexed bacteria monitoring", *Bioconjug. Chem.*, vol. 18, no. 2, pp. 297-301, 2007.
[http://dx.doi.org/10.1021/bc060255n] [PMID: 17341054]

[43] S.A. Kalele, S.S. Ashtaputre, N.Y. Hebalkar, S.W. Gosavi, and D.N. Deobagkar, D.D.D eobagkar, S.K. Kulkarni, "Optical detection of antibody using silica–silver core–shell particles", *Chem. Phys. Lett.*, vol. 404, pp. 136-141, 2005.
[http://dx.doi.org/10.1016/j.cplett.2005.01.064]

[44] E.E. Greciano, B. Matarranz, and L. Sánchez, "Pathway complexity *versus* hierarchical self-assembly in n-annulated perylenes: structural effects in seeded supramolecular polymerization", *Angew. Chem. Int. Ed. Engl.*, vol. 57, no. 17, pp. 4697-4701, 2018.
[http://dx.doi.org/10.1002/anie.201801575] [PMID: 29474002]

[45] S. Nie, D.T. Chiu, and R.N. Zare, "Probing individual molecules with confocal fluorescence microscopy", *Science*, vol. 266, no. 5187, pp. 1018-1021, 1994.
[http://dx.doi.org/10.1126/science.7973650] [PMID: 7973650]

[46] P. Zamora-Perez, D. Tsoutsi, R. Xu, and P. Rivera Gil, "Hyperspectral-enhanced dark field

microscopy for single and collective nanoparticle characterization in biological environments", *Materials (Basel),* vol. 11, no. 2, pp. 1-13, 2018.
[http://dx.doi.org/10.3390/ma11020243] [PMID: 29415420]

[47]   A.L. Lereu, A. Passian, and P. Dumas, "Near field optical microscopy: a brief review", *Int. J. Nanotechnol.,* vol. 9, pp. 3-7, 2012.
[http://dx.doi.org/10.1504/IJNT.2012.045353]

[48]   J. N. A. Matthews, "Commercial optical traps emerge from biophysics labs", *Physics Today,* vol. 62,2, no. 26, pp. 26-27, 2009.

[49]   E. Abbe, *Archiv Microskop. Anat.,* vol. 9, p. 413, 1873.
[http://dx.doi.org/10.1007/BF02956173]

[50]   D. Axelrod, "Selective imaging of surface fluorescence with very high aperture microscope objectives", *J. Biomed. Opt.,* vol. 6, no. 1, pp. 6-13, 2001.
[http://dx.doi.org/10.1117/1.1335689] [PMID: 11178575]

[51]   R.P.J. Barretto, B. Messerschmidt, and M.J. Schnitzer, "*In vivo* fluorescence imaging with high-resolution microlenses", *Nat. Methods,* vol. 6, no. 7, pp. 511-512, 2009.
[http://dx.doi.org/10.1038/nmeth.1339] [PMID: 19525959]

[52]   B. Huang, F. Yu, and R. N. Zare, *Anal. Chem,* vol. 79,7, pp. 2979-2983, 2007.

[53]   B. Huang, M. Bates, and X. Zhuang, "Super-resolution fluorescence microscopy", *Annu. Rev. Biochem.,* vol. 78, pp. 993-1016, 2009.
[http://dx.doi.org/10.1146/annurev.biochem.77.061906.092014] [PMID: 19489737]

[54]   J. Adler, A.I. Shevchuk, P. Novak, Y.E. Korchev, and I. Parmryd, "Plasma membrane topography and interpretation of single-particle tracks", *Nat. Methods,* vol. 7, no. 3, pp. 170-171, 2010.
[http://dx.doi.org/10.1038/nmeth0310-170] [PMID: 20195248]

[55]   I. Parmryd, and B. Onfelt, "Consequences of membrane topography", *FEBS J.,* vol. 280, no. 12, pp. 2775-2784, 2013.
[http://dx.doi.org/10.1111/febs.12209] [PMID: 23438106]

[56]   H.J. Chung, C.M. Castro, H. Im, H. Lee, and R. Weissleder, "A magneto-DNA nanoparticle system for rapid detection and phenotyping of bacteria", *Nat. Nanotechnol.,* vol. 8, no. 5, pp. 369-375, 2013.
[http://dx.doi.org/10.1038/nnano.2013.70] [PMID: 23644570]

[57]   B. Osmani, T. Töpper, and B. Müller, "Conducting and stretchable nanometer-thin gold/thiol-functionalized polydimethylsiloxane films", *J. Nanophoton,* vol. 12,13, no. 033006, pp. 1-11, 2018.

[58]   C. Chen, X. Hou, and J. Si, "Design of a multi-analyte resonant photonic platform for label-free biosensing", *Nanotechnology,* vol. 30, no. 27, p. 275501, 2019.
[http://dx.doi.org/10.1088/1361-6528/ab0771] [PMID: 30769338]

CHAPTER 6

In-Flow Methodologies

Abstract: In-flow methodologies have allowed the development of less time-consuming analytical techniques requiring small volumes of real samples based on microfluidic channels, microfluidic and nanofluidic devices coupled to different optical setups. Moreover, these in-flow systems have led to the confinement of varied nanostructures and functions. Thus, from multifunctional nanoparticles to labelled biostructures, depending on the coupled detection systems, varied signals could be recorded. Likewise, chemical reactions and surface modifications could be developed looking for targeted functional modifications within in-flow methodologies. Accordingly, the detection of single molecules on lab-on particles to single targeted nanostructures, microparticles, bacteria and cells could be recorded from new modes of imaging generated from the control of molecules, surfaces and nanostructures within in flow nano- and micro-channels. Chemical surface modifications could also lead to additional physical sites of interactions and property coupling for real time biosensing.

Keywords: Coupled optical setups, Cytometry, In-flow methodologies, Microfluidic chips, Microfluidics, Nanofluidics.

1. IN-FLOW METHODOLOGIES, MICRO- AND NANOFLUIDIC CHIPS

The aim of this section was to show, based on recent microfluidic developments, how the design of versatile micro- and nanodevices could be incorporated into new advanced clinical research for future nanomedicine treatments [1]. These developments include the nanoscale control for applications such as nanophotonics, genomics, biophotonics and drug delivery studies, along with enhanced imaging resolutions and faster diagnosis and treatments (Fig. **1**) coupled with in-flow methodologies.

In addition, these confined volumes could be chemically modified in order to design functional surfaces with variable physical and chemical properties. Hence, these surfaces within in-flow techniques could provide sites of i) bioconjugations, ii) nano-labelling, iii) chemical reactions, iv) covalent and non-covalent molecular linking, vi) optical interactions and signal transductions from deposed nano-platforms, vii) single nanospectroscopy for chemical sensing, and further types of strategies. Such applications can be potentially used in the controlled contact of low volume of solutions, colloidal dispersions, with modified micro- and nano-surfaces. Thus, they are key variables that could only be overcome by in flow techniques and methods with the appropriate targeted functional nanoplatform.

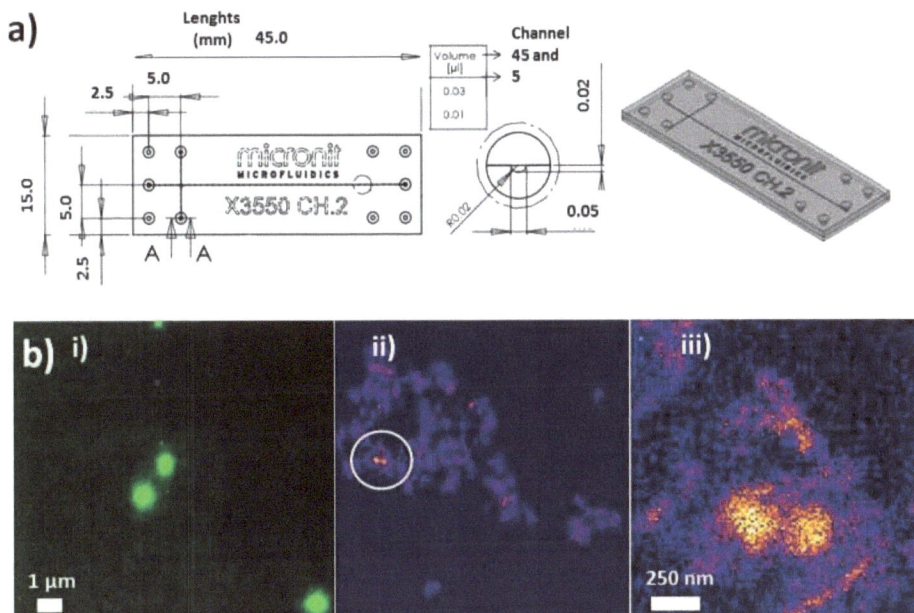

Fig. (1). a) Scheme of cross-channel microfluidic chip. **b)** Inset images correspond to (i) ultraluminescent gold core-shell silica NPs and (ii) and (iii) modified silica nanoparticles with supramolecular systems such as mimetics of antibody antigen interactions for targeted laser fluorescent dyes complexations and detection by laser fluorescence microscopy. Reprinted with permission from A. G. Bracamonte *et al.* Copyright 2019 Frontiers in Drug, Chemistry and Clinical Research, Open Access Text [1].

2. IN-FLOW CYTOMETRY AND MICROFLUIDICS

In-flow methodologies such as cytometry and imaging cytometry [2] were adopted in cell counting and biostructure discrimination, and even in immune-phenotyping to trigger signal processing [3]. This available instrumentation in research and clinical laboratories showed to be an important tool in biochemistry as well. However, enhanced detection approaches are of common interest based on the combination of targeted multifunctional nanoparticles and in-flow methodologies. In this way, the possibility to track nano-biostructures such as virus and genomes could be explored. For this reason the development of new methodologies within in-flow techniques showed to be very/particularly versatile in Life Sciences.

Thus, these techniques were applied when the evaluation of illness caused by pathogens required an accelerated development of point-of-care serological assays with minimal sample volume, low number of manipulations and low cost, as in the rapid and fully microfluidic Ebola virus detection with CRISPR-Cas13a [4]. Here, an automated microfluidic mixing system was combined with a RNA-guided RNA endonuclease Cas13a, integrated with a fluorometer. The enzymatic essay afforded cleaved RNA that, after being automated in flow mixing and fluorescent labelled hybridization, allowed measuring, by fluorescence, low concentrations of specific targeted segments of RNA. Thus, through a 5-min analysis, limits of detections of 20 pfu/ml ($5,45x10^7$ copies.mL^{-1}) of purified Ebola RNA were achieved. Hence, the versatile characteristic of in-flow techniques was combined with high sensitivity detection, enabling faster detections within a low interval of RNA concentrations without amplification. This approach could therefore be transferred to other types of developments based on the combination of controlled key components to conceive new optical in-flow set-ups. Alternatively, numerous advanced standard techniques could be developed and made available on the market for different uses.

In-flow methodologies such as cytometry showed to be very/particularly useful for cell and bacteria detection and biological event tracking. However, the incorporation of imaging systems showed a greater degree of analysis and data recording. Yet, the incorporation of the optimized optical lens within in-flow cytometry systems coupled to cameras for imaging recording has allowed single nanoparticle tracking and small nanoaggregates formed by a few nanoparticles' analysis. On the basis of this enhanced resolution imaging flow cytometry (IFC) experimental set-up, as in genomic applications, the SRY gene, related to sex-genre determination, was detected [5]. Moreover, a PCR-free blood group genotyping was evaluated in real samples using the **FRET-MEF** coupling strategy by the application of the IFC set-up [6]. Thus, in addition to the performance of the nanobiosensor, it was introduced to new PCR-free technologies and to the next generation of sequencing (NGS) methods. In this way, the control of parameters that are still being a challenge in bio-analytical methodologies and NGS was attained. A low time-consuming method was achieved with reduced costs per assay, for non-amplified DNA detection by enhanced signaling.

In this manner, in-flow video and images of single nanoplatforms and microparticles could be recorded. Then, from the single recorded particles, accurate high-sensitivity biosensing information could be gained by tracking signaling between the interacting single targeted DNA aptamers with a modified optical responsive material. This concept of nano platform design could be transferred to other techniques, chemical modifications, bioconjugations and physical phenomena. In addition, in all these new set-ups, new variables to evaluate should be defined considering the different scales of the in-flow channels. New in-flow methodologies are in progress, including microfluidics and nanofluidics coupled to advanced optical instrumentation. These reduced-size channels of few micro- to nanometre diameters and millimetres have allowed the synthesis and incorporation of reduced-size nanoparticles within confined volumes for enhanced resolution. Different techniques have been developed for microfluidic design. [7]. Soft lithography and PDMS (polydimethylsiloxane) are among the most widely applied techniques and materials in use, respectively. However, many other organic polymers and hybrid layer deposition have also been used in view of specific needs and applications. In this sense, lower-volume channels were designed and combined with varied bonding techniques. Studies reported size ranging from few to hundreds of micrometers and variable designs from crossing channels to multi-channel chips, on silanized substrates of few cm^2 surfaces, with varied volume for different residence time of fluids. Thus, going through these channels was possible with, for instance, few microliters (μL) such as 2.0-5.0 μL intervals per varied and controlled period of time. On the basis of these chips, many applications were reported, such as these microdevices with micropumps and optical detection systems coupled to or incorporated in standard commercial instrumentation and in-flow cytometry. In addition, we should note the extension of these in-flow systems to other types of technological developments, such as the incorporation of Ferrobotic system in automated microfluidic systems for weareable, automated and tactile responsive materials [8].

Automated technologies that can add extra functionalities and properties, such as remote guided vehicle systems on the micro- and nanoscales, could lead to advanced approaches of micro- and nanofluidic manipulations based on targeted tasks in cooperation with other functional components. Thus, different material properties could be combined toward a functional device. The magnetic properties could be used as a driven force within in-flow systems that, in conjunction with an appropriate bioconjugation, could produce collaborative tasks, as in biomarkers detections and separations. Consequently it is important to note the synthesis of nanoparticles with different physical properties within confined spaces with minimal volumes of reactants [9], bioanalytical flow cells for biofilm studies [10], microfluidic flow confinement to avoid chemotaxis-based upstream growth [11] and bioanalytical applications such as biostructure counting [12] and biological event detection [13]. Yet, reduction of even smaller volumes was required for highly accurate optical nanomaterial characterization and improved resolution for tracking of individual events, favoring developments in fluidics on the nanoscale.

In this respect, based on the combination of intrinsic nanomaterial properties incorporated into in-flow systems, we could put forward innovative solutions such as the PCR-Free DNA detection using a magnetic bead-supported polymeric transducer and microelectromagnetic traps [14]. In this approach, the DNA was directly targeted on magnetic particles as probes joined with a fluorescent polymer intercalating agent. Hence, in presence of the complementary targeted DNA sequence, the intercaled polymer modified its configuration from a planar to an anti-planar structure, showing an increase in fluorescence signal. This increased fluorescence signaling generated only in the presence of the complentary double stranded DNA led to the detection event of the targeted DNA. This detection event was recorded within confined volumes in a magnetic trap, allowing improved performance by reducing pre-concentration steps and separations.

3. NANOFLLUIDICS

Highly accurate methodologies to develop in-flow channels on the nanoscale have been reported. The development of nanofluidic devices has involved dimensions below 100.0 nm, and therefore, lower volumes were applied in the methodologies developed. It was also possible to work with higher volumes and surface ratios from individual nanoarchitectures or small nanoaggregates where chemical interactions and new properties on short length scales have aroused increasing interest [15]. That is the case of studies on nano-optics in low volumes for individual nanoparticle analysis and tracking for real-time plasmonic lasing from nanocavity arrays incorporated into nanochannels (Fig. **2**) [16].

Note, in addition, that the tuning of these confined volumes on these scales of intervals has allowed achieving molecular events, molecular transport and detection in close proximity to the site where the physical or chemical modification occurs. In this way, the development of nanofluidic structures for coupled functionalities such as sensing and remediation of toxins could be carried out [17]. In addition, signal recording was performed on varied scales, from quantum in-flow signaling [18] to higher size nanostructure property tracking. Thus, a nano flow cytometer for single lipid vesicle analysis was developed [19]. This nanofluidic device consisted in parallel nanochannels with a square profile of 300 nm connected by two micro-channels used for injections. Thus, time lapse movies allowed the detection and counting of modified vesicles with fluorescent reporters with an epi-fluorescence microscope.

These in-flow confined volume approaches are feasible with low-volume use, fast detection and tracking and low costs since small reagent quantities are required. In addition, their relatively easy accessibility to the design of your own in-flow chips via kits provided by commercial companies increases the possibility of furthering studies. For example, from genomics, available DNA detection boxes for forensic applications have been offered by widely known and important companies promoting legal debates. Hence, we are only in the beginning of an increasingly fertile research field with high science, industry and social impact.

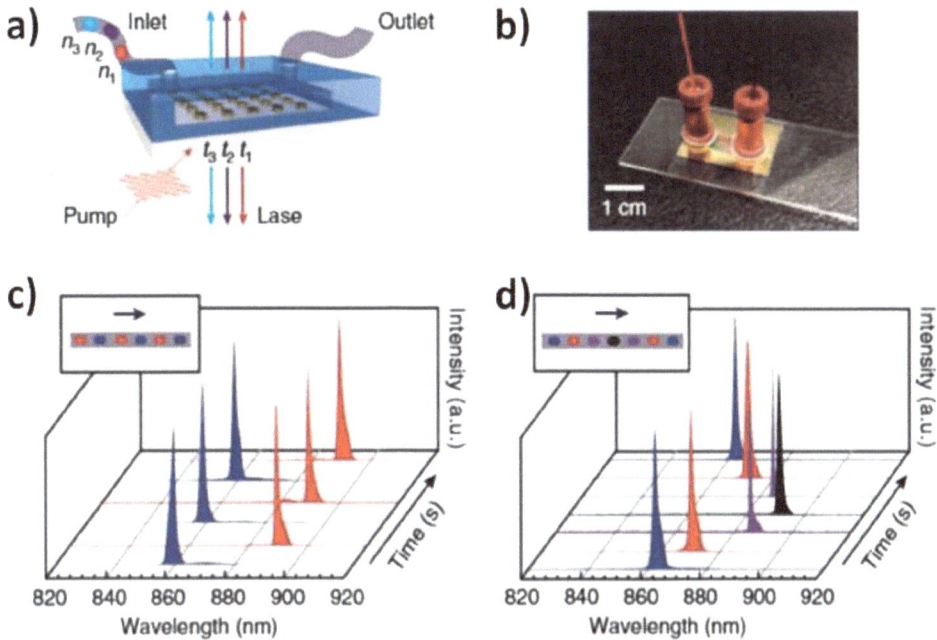

Fig. (2). Lasing emissions from Au nanoparticle arrays in real time. **a)** Scheme of the dynamic laser; **b)** photograph of the device; **c)** switching lasing wavelengths and; **d)** shifting lasing wavelengths. Note: In c, IR-140 dye molecules were dissolved in DMSO (blue) and BA (red). In d, IR-140 dye molecules were dissolved in DMSO (blue), DMSO:BA=2:1 (red), DMSO: BA=1:2 (purple) and BA (black). DMSO:dimethyl sulfoxide, BA: benzyl alcohol. The emission intensities were normalized [16].

CONCLUDING REMARKS

The development of different types and designs of in-flow chips based on different materials for a wide range of applications has opened up new research fields related to the confinement of molecules, biomolecules, nanostructures and biostructures for advanced studies on the interaction and generation of new modes of detection, according to coupled optical setups. These fundamental studies have produced commercial kits and portable instrumentation, challenging standardized methodology.

Moreover, this ability of the control of fluidics on different scales and volumes could track phenomena from molecular events, nanoparticles, nanoplatforms with close proximity to quantum events depending on the optical set-ups used. Then, higher size nanoplatforms and biostructures, ranging from vesicles to bacteria and cells, could be tracked. In this manner, the detection could be achieved with a single step through complex mechanisms, where non-classical light pathways and functionalities occurred below the nanoscale; as discussed along this chapter.

REFERENCES

[1]   C. Salinas, and A.G. Bracamonte, "From microfluidics to nanofluidics and signal wave-guiding for nanophotonics, biophotonics resolution and drug delivery, frontiers in drug", *Chemistry and Clinical Research,* vol. 2, pp. 1-6, 2019.

[2]   N.S. Barteneva, E. Fasler-Kan, and I.A. Vorobjev, "Imaging flow cytometry: coping with heterogeneity in biological systems", *J. Histochem. Cytochem.,* vol. 60, no. 10, pp. 723-733, 2012. [http://dx.doi.org/10.1369/0022155412453052] [PMID: 22740345]

[3]   P. Lin, R. Owens, G. Tricot, and C.S. Wilson, "Flow cytometric immunophenotypic analysis of 306 cases of multiple myeloma", *Am. J. Clin. Pathol.,* vol. 121, no. 4, pp. 482-488, 2004. [http://dx.doi.org/10.1309/74R4TB90BUWH27JX] [PMID: 15080299]

[4]   P. Qin, M. Park, K.J. Alfson, M. Tamhankar, R. Carrion, J.L. Patterson, A. Griffiths, Q. He, A. Yildiz, R. Mathies, and K. Du, "Rapid and Fully Microfluidic Ebola Virus Detection with CRISPR-Cas13a", *ACS Sens.,* vol. 4, no. 4, pp. 1048-1054, 2019. [http://dx.doi.org/10.1021/acssensors.9b00239] [PMID: 30860365]

[5]   D. Brouard, O. Ratelle, A.G. Bracamonte, M. St-Louis, and D. Boudreau, "Direct molecular detection of SRY gene from unamplified genomic DNA by metal enhanced fluorescence and FRET", *Anal. Methods,* vol. 5, pp. 6896-6899, 2013. [http://dx.doi.org/10.1039/c3ay41428k]

[6]   D. Brouard, O. Ratelle, J. Perreault, D. Boudreau, and M. St-Louis, "PCR-free blood group genotyping using a nanobiosensor", *Vox Sang.,* vol. 108, no. 2, pp. 197-204, 2015. [http://dx.doi.org/10.1111/vox.12207] [PMID: 25469570]

[7]   M. Leester-Schadel, T. Lorenz, F. Jurgens, and C. Richter, *Fabrication of Microfluidics Devices, Microsystems for Pharmatechnology* Springer International Publishing: Switzerland A, 2016.

[8]   W. Yu, H. Lin, Y. Wang, X. He, N. Chen, K. Sun, D. Lo, B. Cheng, C. Yeung, J. Tan, D. Di Cario, and S. Emaminejad, "A Ferrobotic system for automated microfluidic logistics", *Sci. Robotics,* vol. 5, pp. 1-11, 2020. [PMID: eaba4411]

[9]   W. Li, J. Greener, D. Voicu, and E. Kumacheva, "Multiple modular microfluidic (M3) reactors for the synthesis of polymer particles", *Lab Chip,* vol. 9, no. 18, pp. 2715-2721, 2009. [http://dx.doi.org/10.1039/b906626h] [PMID: 19704988]

[10]   M. Pousti, M. Zarabadi, and M.A. Amirdehi, F. Paquet -Mercier, and J. Greener, "Microfluidic bioanalytical flow cells for biofilm studies: A review", *Analyst (Lond.),* vol. 144, pp. 68-86, 2019. [http://dx.doi.org/10.1039/C8AN01526K]

[11]   F. Asayesh, M.P. Zarabadi, N.B. Aznaveh, and J. Greener, "Microfluidic flow confinement to avoid chemotaxis-based upstream growth in a biofilm flow cell reactor", *Anal. Methods,* vol. 10, pp. 4579-4587, 2018. [http://dx.doi.org/10.1039/C8AY01513A]

[12]   S.-Yi Yang, S.-K.Hsiung, Y.-C. Hung, C.-M.Chang, T.-L. Liao, and G.-B. Lee, "A cell counting/sorting system incorporated with a microfabricated flow cytometer chip", *Meas. Sci. Technol.,* vol. 17, pp. 2001-2009, 2006. [http://dx.doi.org/10.1088/0957-0233/17/7/045]

[13]   J. Skommer, J. Akagi, K. Takeda, Y. Fujimura, K. Khoshmanesh, and D. Wlodkowic, "Multiparameter Lab-on-a-Chip flow cytometry of the cell cycle", *Biosens. Bioelectron.,* vol. 42, pp. 586-591, 2013. [http://dx.doi.org/10.1016/j.bios.2012.11.008] [PMID: 23261693]

[14]   S. Dubus, J.F. Gravel, B. Le Drogoff, P. Nobert, T. Veres, and D. Boudreau, "PCR-free DNA detection using a magnetic bead-supported polymeric transducer and microelectromagnetic traps", *Anal. Chem.,* vol. 78, no. 13, pp. 4457-4464, 2006.
[http://dx.doi.org/10.1021/ac060486n] [PMID: 16808454]

[15]   C. Duan, W. Wang, and Q. Xie, "Review article: Fabrication of nanofluidic devices", *Biomicrofluidics,* vol. 7, no. 2, p. 26501, 2013.
[http://dx.doi.org/10.1063/1.4794973] [PMID: 23573176]

[16]   A. Yang, T.B. Hoang, M. Dridi, C. Deeb, M.H. Mikkelsen, G.C. Schatz, and T.W. Odom, "Real-time tunable lasing from plasmonic nanocavity arrays", *Nat. Commun.,* vol. 6, no. 6939, p. 6939, 2015.
[http://dx.doi.org/10.1038/ncomms7939] [PMID: 25891212]

[17]   K. Shaw, N.M. Contento, W. Xu, and P.W. Bohn, "Nanofluidic structures for coupled sensing and remediation of toxins, Proc. SPIE,9107", *Smart Biomedical and Physiological Sensor Technology XI,* vol. 91070L, pp. 1-11, 2014.

[18]   P.D. Hislop, K. Kirkpatrick, S. Olla, and J. Schenker, "Transport of a quantum particle in a time dependent white noise potential", *J. Math. Phys.,* vol. 60, no. 083303, pp. 1-12, 2019.
[http://dx.doi.org/10.1063/1.5054017]

[19]   R. Friedrich, S. Block, M. Alizadehheidari, S. Heider, J. Fritzsche, E.K. Esbjörner, F. Westerlund, and M. Bally, "A nano flow cytometer for single lipid vesicle analysis", *Lab Chip,* vol. 17, no. 5, pp. 830-841, 2017.
[http://dx.doi.org/10.1039/C6LC01302C] [PMID: 28128381]

CHAPTER 7

Signal Detection Waveguiding

Abstract: Signal Waveguiding successfully diminished signal loss for routing different types and modes of energy, based on the optimization of energy transfer in confined channels or patterned surfaces where signal routing occurred through planar surfaces. For these reasons, all the modifications of well-known dielectric materials that enhanced signals of different wavelengths generated different types of waveguides, such as silica waveguides, organic waveguides and hybrid waveguides. In addition, from enhanced plasmonic signals, plasmonic waveguides were developed by combining and coupling different nanomaterials and metamaterials.

Keywords: Hybrid materials for waveguiding, Metamaterials for waveguides, Organic waveguide, Photon and quantum signal transduction, Plasmonic waveguiding, Signal waveguiding, Silica waveguide.

1. INTRODUCTION

The detection of signal, from communication to sensing applications, still poses a major challenge since a signal loss has awakened special interest in enhanced signal approaches [1]. Silicon photonics showed to be largely applied to different microdevice fabrications. These devices were based on the intrinsic properties of silicon related to optical transparent properties and semi-conductive characteristics in controlled conditions, for instance, silica waveguides such as modified silica surfaces to conduct signals within confined channels. With this type of device, signal transduction occurred through planar-modified surfaces; thus, the transduction of detected light signals of targeted wavelengths generated from the nanoscale could be transmitted through millimeter lengths.

2. MATERIALS USED FOR WAVEGUIDE FABRICATIONS

In order to avoid signal loss, modification of silicon channels with different conductive materials should be considered, in view of the targeted signals and the design of the signal guiding and routing. In relation to fabrication and modification of silica waveguides, we could also consider new metamaterials developed through resonant plasmonic approaches with core-shell nanoparticles for fluorescence signal routing potentially applied to biomolecular sensing in microdevices [2]. In addition, these metamaterials used for silica waveguides also have a major influence on studies of quantum optical circuits, where routing and detection of resonance fluorescence could be applied, as it was reported recently on-chips [3].

The modification of silica waveguides with different materials has led to different types of wave routing, as reported recently in the strongly confined surface plasmon polariton wave guiding achieved by planar staggered plasmonic waveguides [4]. In this sense, signal transductions and detections were observed in the far field from electromagnetic fields generated by laser excitation in the near field of metallic surfaces within silica waveguides. These research approaches to advanced signal Waveguiding are in progress in search of potential high-impact applications for new analytical and bioanalytical methodologies. Then, the incorporation of graphene as an organic conductor in waveguides showed a high sensitive plasmonic resonance Waveguiding [5]. In particular, growing interest has been shown in graphene as a nanomaterial to be incorporated into waveguides due to its electronic and semi-conductive properties, allowing, from modified substrates with different thickness, periodic control by voltage modulation of their bands coupled to plasmonics for band rejection applications.

In this Research field, the design of new metamaterials showed to be highly required in signal transductions. For example, long-range dipole-dipole interactions were observed in hyperbolic metamaterials consisting of Waveguide platforms based on hybrid donor-acceptor emitters deposed on silica-metallic nanoarrays [6].

3. APPLICATIONS

Since the design of these novel metamaterials, new modes of signal transduction applied to different research fields are in progress, as well as their incorporation in new high technological devices. New analytical approaches and methodologies include those based on ultrasensitive resonant photonic waveguides, label-free biosensing and signal propagation and transduction taking place in one dimension in patterned waveguides, were applied through microfluidic channels [7]. In this manner, it was placed in contact with the conductive modified surfaces for the fabrication of standard spectroscopical instrumentation commercially available at present. For example, the spectroscopic technique, known as optical Waveguide lightmode spectroscopy (OWLS), which could be used from in-flow surface characterization studies [8] to cell and molecular detection [9] and adsorption of proteins [10].

CONCLUDING REMARKS

From the different examples described, it should be highlighted that for efficient signal transduction through planar surfaces the type and mode of energy to be transferred for the development of the required material should be considered. The strategy is then applied for the enhanced signal Waveguiding. Therefore, it was fabricated from micro-waveguide chips to optical waveguide lightmode spectroscopy known as WOLS, enabling the detection of proteins based on chemical surface modification with fluorescence resonance routing from quantum particles. Signal Waveguiding also demonstrated to be the basis of different types of energy routing through optical and quantum circuits.

REFERENCES

[1]   C. Salinas, and A.G. Bracamonte, "From microfluidics to nanofluidics and signal wave-guiding for nanophotonics, biophotonics resolution and drug delivery, frontiers in drug", *Chemistry and Clinical Research,* vol. 2, pp. 1-6, 2019.

[2]   A. Grégoire, and D. Boudreau, "Chapter 28: Metal-Enhanced Fluorescence in Plasmonic Waveguides", *Nano-Optics: Principles Enabling Basic Research and Applications, NATO Science for Peace and Security Series B: Physics and Biophysics,* Springer Science+Business Media Dordrecht, 2017.

[3]   G. Reithmaier, M. Kaniber, F. Flassig, S. Lichtmannecker, K. Müller, A. Andrejew, J. Vučković, R. Gross, and J.J. Finley, "On-chip generation, routing, and detection of resonance fluorescence", *Nano Lett.,* vol. 15, no. 8, pp. 5208-5213, 2015.
[http://dx.doi.org/10.1021/acs.nanolett.5b01444] [PMID: 26102603]

[4]   L. Ye, Y. Xiao, Y. Liu, L. Zhang, G. Cai, and Q.H. Liu, "Strongly confined spoof surface plasmon polaritons waveguiding enabled by planar staggered plasmonic waveguides", *Sci. Rep.,* vol. 6, no. 38528, p. 38528, 2016.
[http://dx.doi.org/10.1038/srep38528] [PMID: 27917930]

[5]   M. Azar, and Y. Zehforoosh, "Periodically voltage modulated graphene plasmonic waveguide for band rejection applications", *J. Nanophotonics,* vol. 12, no. 4, pp. 1-2, 2018.
[http://dx.doi.org/10.1117/1.JNP.12.046002]

[6]   W. D. Newman, C. L. Cortes, A. Afshar, K. Cadien, A. Afshar, K. Cadien, A. Meldrum, R. Fedosejevs, and Z. Jacob, "Observation of long range dipole dipole interactions in hyperbolic metamaterials", *Science Advances,* vol. 4, no. eaar5278, pp. 1-7, 2018.

[7]   F. Dell'Olio, D. Conteduca, C. Ciminelli, and M.N. Armenise, "New ultrasensitive resonant photonic platform for label-free biosensing", *Opt. Express,* vol. 23, no. 22, pp. 28593-28604, 2015.
[http://dx.doi.org/10.1364/OE.23.028593] [PMID: 26561129]

[8]   H. Yu, C.M. Eggleston, J. Chen, W. Wang, Q. Dai, and J. Tang, "Optical waveguide lightmode spectroscopy (OWLS) as a sensor for thin film and quantum dot corrosion", *Sensors (Basel),* vol. 12, no. 12, pp. 17330-17342, 2012.
[http://dx.doi.org/10.3390/s121217330] [PMID: 23443400]

[9]   R.C. Gunawan, J.A. King, B.P. Lee, P.B. Messersmith, and W.M. Miller, "Surface presentation of bioactive ligands in a nonadhesive background using DOPA-tethered biotinylated poly(ethylene glycol)", *Langmuir,* vol. 23, no. 21, pp. 10635-10643, 2007.
[http://dx.doi.org/10.1021/la701415z] [PMID: 17803326]

[10]   J. Vörös, "The density and refractive index of adsorbing protein layers", *Biophys. J.,* vol. 87, no. 1, pp. 553-561, 2004.
[http://dx.doi.org/10.1529/biophysj.103.030072] [PMID: 15240488]

CHAPTER 8

Design of Nano and Micro-devices

Abstract: For the design and fabrication of nano- and microdevices, a set of different techniques should be available for the control of both scales, as discussed previously, from wet-chemistry synthetic methodologies to lithography techniques by the application of high-energy lasers and electron beam excitations. Recent developments in the field have already been introduced and discussed in the previous chapters, showing the control of the nanoscale to higher dimensions. In the examples, varied and controlled physical properties such as magnetism, plasmonics, conduction and energy transfer were applied, coupled to the right tuning of chemically modified and nano-patterned surfaces incorporated into devices of varied dimensions. Moreover, these devices should be combined with different optical setups for excitation and detection for specific functions. Consequently, interdisciplinary knowledge should be gained so as to meet innovation challenges with improved performance.

Keywords: Lab-on chips, Light emitter devices (**LEDs**), Microdevices, Nanodevices, Optical traps, Waveguides.

1. DESIGN AND FABRICATION OF LAB-ON PARTICLES AND CHIPS

Based on the properties of nanomaterials already referred to, properties in the nanoscale could be tuned to design nanoplatforms, such as free functional nanodevices used as nanotools. They could be incorporated into microdevices as part of constitutive material or into nano- and micro-fluidic channels. In addition, these components could be part of advanced instrumentation, where multidisciplinary fields are involved.

For example, for the control of the nanoscale, chemical surface modification was combined with lithography techniques in in-flow channels to develop multimodal technologies based on hybrid nanomaterials with magnetic and fluorescent properties for biosensing applications. Therefore, PCR-Free DNA detection microdevices were designed incorporating magnetic bead-supported polymeric transducer in in-flow microelectromagnetic traps [1]. These reduced-size microdevices were based on grafted "target-ready" microbeads modified with a fluorescent poly-thiophene polymer and suitable DNA probe. Thus, enhanced fluorescence signals were recorded in the presence of the complementary targeted DNA strands from the grafted beads collected by a micro-electromagnetic trap within a confined cavity, also coupled to optical detection. This microdevice offered a pre-concentration step coupled to a dual-mode of detection in the same support.

This is also the case in lab-on-a-disc agglutination assay for protein detection by optomagnetic readout and optical imaging, using nano- and micro-sized magnetic beads [2]. The detection of these lab-on particles resulted from aptamer-coated magnetic microbeads that, in the presence of Thrombin, varied microaggregation was recorded according to concentration levels. Protein agglutination was induced *via* the application of strong magnetic field pulses within the modified magnetic bead colloidal dispersion, and their detection was done by an optomagnetic readout and optical imaging. An integrated and automated, low-cost microfluidic disc platform was devised with minimal manual steps involved.

Light emitter devices (**LEDs**) represent a further example from molecular-level research, leading to a higher level of design and engineering of reduced-size devices for targeted applications. From the appropriate tuning of donor-acceptor molecular emitter pair, optimal electroluminescent properties were studied by electro-stimuli-responsive materials [3] potentially incorporated in color-tunable emitters in organic light-emitting diodes (**OLEDs**). There, a stimuli-responsive fluorophoric molecular system was reported capable of switching their **OLEDs** emission colors between green and orange in the solid-state. The incorporation of secondary optical components such as metallic nanostructures for improved efficiency **LED** lighting [4] known as plasmonic light emitter devices (**P-LEDs**) and plasmonic organic light emitter devices (**P-OLEDs**), is also worth mentioning. For instance, the incorporation of aluminium nanoparticles covered with a red dye layer was carried out to develop enhanced emitter devices. Aluminium nanocylinders of 140 nm, along with thin luminescent layered material, have allowed recording thin resonances with improvements ranging from 70 and 20 with blue laser excitation and Lambertian LED, respectively [5]. Their use and incorporation in advanced instrumentation at different scales are particularly significant, from smaller devices for neuronal excitation [6] and incorporation in flexible patches [7] requiring light stimulation to artificial intelligence and decision taken, as in autonomous drive [8].

As discussed previously, we need to underline the importance of signal transduction and routing in devices to develop waveguides and their incorporation into on-chips for different applications. Cases include metal-enhanced fluorescence resonance modes by incorporating core-shell nanoarchitectures in silica plasmonic waveguides, direct on-chip optical plasmon detection through an atomically thin $IMoS_2$ wire semiconductor [9] and by the use of quantum-dots on-chips *via* semi-conductive GaAs ridge waveguides for routing and detection of resonance fluorescence.

As evident, from the accurate control of the nanoscale for the nanoarchitecture, it was possible to design, test and apply different approaches. At this order of lengths, the controlled positions of the different parts of the micro- and nano-devices were essentials for optimal performances.

In relation to miniaturization, rapid sensing and diagnosis, monolithically integrated mid-infrared lab-on-a-chip was designed using plasmonic and quantum cascade structures [10]. This microdevice was devised on a monolithically integrated sensor based on mid-infrared absorption spectroscopy. A bi-functional quantum cascade laser/detector was used, whereby changing the applied bias, the device switched between laser and detector operation, while the chemical sensing was within a dielectric-loaded surface plasmon polariton waveguide. The thin dielectric layer enhanced the confinement and enabled efficient end-fire coupling from and to the laser and detector (Fig. **1**).

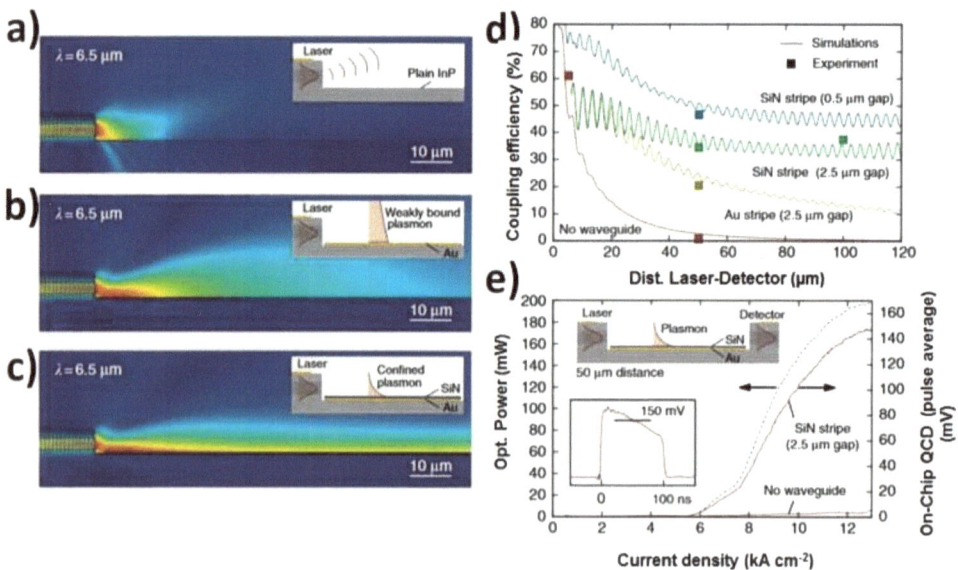

Fig. (**1**). **a)** Without waveguide light couples to free space and partially into the substrate. **b)** An SPP can be excited on the gold surface, but is weakly bound to the interface. **c)** The 200-nm-thick SiNx layer on top of the gold surface leads to increased confinement. Owing to high confinement, this SPP can be coupled directly to a detector. **d)** Coupling efficiency from the laser to detector facet over the distance between them, with the simulation as curves and the experiment as points. **e)** Detector signal into 50O compared with the laser power (front facet) over the laser current density for a distance of 50mm. The inset shows the time-resolved detector signal [10].

On-chip spectroscopy [11, 12] can also be considered for spontaneous parametric down-conversion (SPDC) spectroscopy, performing mid-infrared (mid-IR) spectroscopy without the need for dedicated sources and detectors in the mid-IR which can be expensive and limited in performance, which consists of an integrated on-chip version using lithium niobate waveguides. In this respect, the implementation of molecular bottom-up approaches and nanostructures with controlled nanoarchitecture and patterning for specific functional devices has been briefly discussed.

CONCLUDING REMARKS

The design of devices for multiple functionalities showed a high potential from fundamental research to the required applications. Many uses could be highlighted in different areas of interests and requirements. For example, for better human well-being, Real-Time Bio-monitoring is applied for sports and the high point of health care analysis for Precision Medicine, as well as other types of devices from **LEDs** to wearable, uses.

REFERENCES

[1]   S. Dubus, J-F. Gravel, B. Le Drogoff, P. Nobert, T. Veres, and D. Boudreau, "PCR-free DNA detection using a magnetic bead-supported polymeric transducer and microelectromagnetic traps", *Anal. Chem.*, vol. 78, no. 13, pp. 4457-4464, 2006.
[http://dx.doi.org/10.1021/ac060486n] [PMID: 16808454]

[2]   R. Uddin, R. Burger, M. Donolato, J. Fock, M. Creagh, M.F. Hansen, and A. Boisen, "Lab-on-a-disc agglutination assay for protein detection by optomagnetic readout and optical imaging using nano- and micro-sized magnetic beads", *Biosens. Bioelectron.*, vol. 85, pp. 351-357, 2016.
[http://dx.doi.org/10.1016/j.bios.2016.05.023] [PMID: 27183287]

[3]   K. Isayama, N. Aizawa, J.Y. Kim, and T. Yasuda, "Modulating photo- and electroluminescence in a stimuli-responsive π-conjugated donor-acceptor molecular system", *Angew. Chem. Int. Ed. Engl.*, vol. 57, no. 37, pp. 11982-11986, 2018.
[http://dx.doi.org/10.1002/anie.201806863] [PMID: 30039632]

[4]   G. Lozano, S.R.K. Rodriguez, M.A. Verschuuren, and J. Gómez Rivas, "Metallic nanostructures for efficient LED lighting", *Light Sci. Appl.*, vol. 5, no. 6, p. e16080, 2016.
[http://dx.doi.org/10.1038/lsa.2016.80] [PMID: 30167168]

[5]   M. Lunz, D. de Boer, G. Lozano, S.R.K. Rodriguez, J. Gomez Rivas, and M.A. Verschuuren, "Plasmonic LED devices", *SPIE Proceeding,* 2014pp. 1-6
[http://dx.doi.org/] [PMID: 9127N]

[6]   N. Grossman, V. Poher, M.S. Grubb, G.T. Kennedy, K. Nikolic, B. McGovern, and R. Berlinguer, Palmini, Z. Gong, E. M Drakakis, M. A A Neil, M. D Dawson, J. Burrone, and P. Degenaar, "Multi-site optical excitation using ChR2 and micro-LED array", *J. Neural Eng.*, vol. 7, no. 016004, pp. 1-13, 2010.

[7]   M. Choi, Y. Ju Park, B. K. Sharma, S. R. Bae, S. Young Kim, and J. H. Ahn, "Flexible active matrix organic light emitting diode display enabled by MoS2 thin film transistor", *Sci. Adv,* vol. 4, pp. 1-7, 2018.
[PMID: eaas8721]

[8]　S. Chen, "Biomedical Optics & Medical Imaging, Hardwiring the Brain", *SPIE Newsroom (International Society for Optics and Photonics),* 2019.

[9]　K.M. Goodfellow, C. Chakraborty, R. Beams, L. Novotny, and A.N. Vamivakas, "Direct On-Chip Optical Plasmon Detection with an Atomically Thin Semiconductor", *Nano Lett.,* vol. 15, no. 8, pp. 5477-5481, 2015.
[http://dx.doi.org/10.1021/acs.nanolett.5b01898] [PMID: 26120877]

[10]　B. Schwarz, P. Reininger, D. Ristanić, H. Detz, A.M. Andrews, W. Schrenk, and G. Strasser, "Monolithically integrated mid-infrared lab-on-a-chip using plasmonics and quantum cascade structures", *Nat. Commun.,* vol. 5, no. 4085, p. 4085, 2014.
[http://dx.doi.org/10.1038/ncomms5085] [PMID: 24905443]

[11]　"Mid-Infrared Optics on-chip spectroscopy", *APL Photon.,* vol. 3, p. 021301, 2018.

[12]　O. Graydon, "Mid-Infrared Optics, On-chip spectroscopy", *Nat. Photonics,* vol. 12, no. 189, pp. 1-2, 2018.

CHAPTER 9

Nano-optics, Photonic and Quantum Circuits

Abstract: For the design of photonic and quantum circuits, special nanomaterials should be applied in order to transduce controlled quantized types and modes of energy through developed hybrid nanomaterials and metamaterials. Therefore, it is important to discuss the way in which photon delivery could be controlled from developed quantum emitters and nano-optical platforms below the nanoscale, based on energy shuttle to pass through the tuned and patterned material of the designed circuit. In this way, to gain further insights into these phenomena, examples from solar cells to modified photonic surfaces are being discussed, in addition to the generation of energy routing imaging modes.

Keywords: Microelectronics, Nano-optics, Nanophotonics, Photonic circuits, Photovoltaics, Quantics, Quantum circuits, Quantum phenomena.

1. CONCEPTS OF QUANTIZED PHOTON INTERACTIONS WITH NANOMATERIALS

Based on the control of the nanoscale and below, electronic, quantum and plasmonic properties could be tuned having an impact on the conductive properties of the nanomaterials and their incorporation in photonic circuits for multiple applications. These advanced optical systems have allowed different types of studies by the incorporation of high-power irradiance lasers and high-sensitive detectors in highly accurate patterned nanostructured surfaces of different semi-conductive materials. Hence, single-photon counting and conduction and generation of virtual resonance photonic modes in chips have been reported, potentially incorporated to quantum computers and light-responsive devices.

First of all, in order to understand the photonic, quantum circuits, different concepts and issues related to the control of classical and non-classical light, photons and quantum phenomena should be discussed. This level of knowledge has been demonstrated in the frontiers of the nanoscale and below based on different designs, sizes and shapes of nano-patterned materials and metamaterials.

To begin, we should mention the guided-mode resonance of light by grating pattern fabrication on a glass substrate using laser interference lithography followed by a transparent conducting oxide coating as a top contact [1]. A ~320-nm thick p-i-n hydrogenated amorphous silicon (a-Si:H) solar cell was deposited over the patterned substrate followed by bottom contact deposition. Thus, light trapping was demonstrated in thin-film solar cells through guided-mode resonance (GMR) effects. As a result, resonant field enhancement and propagation path elongation led to enhanced solar absorption. Around 35% integrated absorption enhancement was observed over the 450 to 750-nm wavelength range, compared to that found in a planar reference solar cell. From these types of studies, we could observe how surface grating could modify the photon transmission and absorption.

2. PHOTONIC SURFACE MODIFICATIONS

If these conductive materials were modified with accurate atomic layer depositions or with the incorporation of semi-conductive and plasmonic nano-patterned surfaces, light propagation could be highly affected and controlled properties could be obtained, depending on the nanomaterial characteristics added. Therefore, phase-controlled propagation of surface plasmons [2] could be developed from the quantum near field frontiers to the far-field. For example, from a properly shaped single antenna or a phased array of individual antennas, directional emission of electromagnetic radiation could be achieved. In this way, the propagation of surface plasmons at the interface between metal films and dielectric materials can be determined by shaping the individual surface nanostructures or *via* phase control of individual elements in an array of such structures. The fabrication of plasmonic surface propagation that is different on both sides of a metal film provides a unique opportunity for such control. Thus, the design of the patterning is highly important not only for the properties recorded or modified but also for the directional and asymmetrical translation of the signals within circuits.

3. DESIGN OF SUBWAVELENGTH CIRCUITS AND APPLICATIONS

As referred to before, circuits with light at the nanoscale and optical nanocircuits based on metamaterials [3] were obtained by manipulating the local optical electric fields and electric displacement vectors in a subwavelength domain, leading to the possibility of optical information processing at the nanometer scale. By exploiting the optical properties of metamaterials, these nanoparticles may play the role of "lumped" nanocircuit elements such as nanoinductors, nanocapacitors and nanoresistors, analogous to microelectronics. It was shown that this concept of metamaterial-inspired nanoelectronics ("metactronics") can bring the tools and mathematical machinery of the circuit theory into optics, which may link the fields of optics, electronics, plasmonics and metamaterials and provide road maps to future innovations in nanoscale optical devices, components and more intricate nanoscale metamaterials.

Chemically, implications of chemistry and supramolecular chemistry in new optoelectronic metamaterials include the design of nanomesh scaffold for supramolecular nanowire optoelectronic devices [4] and strong coupling superconductivity in a quasiperiodic host-guest structure [5], generating strong electron-photon coupling with potential applications in superconducting materials. These examples showed how the design of functionalized materials by the tuning from the chemical level to the nm and micro-scales, in addition to measureable properties, could be applied also in photonic circuits.

Many research studies report different designs and variables affecting photon conduction within photonic circuits. In this way, 2D dimensional nanomaterials were assayed from larger sizes within the nano-scale, such as 100 nm nano-patterned surfaces to below 5 nm arrays, where quantum-confined phenomena could generate quantum circuits. For instance, sub-2 nm quantum well arrays obtained by tuning quantum well superlattices allowed controllable band alignment and nanoscale widths for interconnective 2D conductive integrated circuits *via* n-type modulation doping [6] (Fig. **1**).

Moreover, quantum information processing requires accuracy in the control of dimensions by logarithmic scale modifications for quantum networks and photonic circuits. However, the incorporation of intermediate excitations between the different components added extra noise and limited bandwidths. Yet, this issue could be solved by incorporating superconducting and optical cavities in the same chip for triple electro-optic resonance generated from the quantized electronic properties below the 1.0 nm scale added [7]. Hence, internal conversion efficiencies of 25%, together with 2.05% of total efficiency, were recorded. These studies offered potential applications toward integrated hybrid quantum circuits. Additionally, the incorporation of rare earth minerals has allowed the development of electronic devices as well as their use in nanophotonic research, such as nanophotonic rare-earth quantum memory with optically controlled retrieval [8].

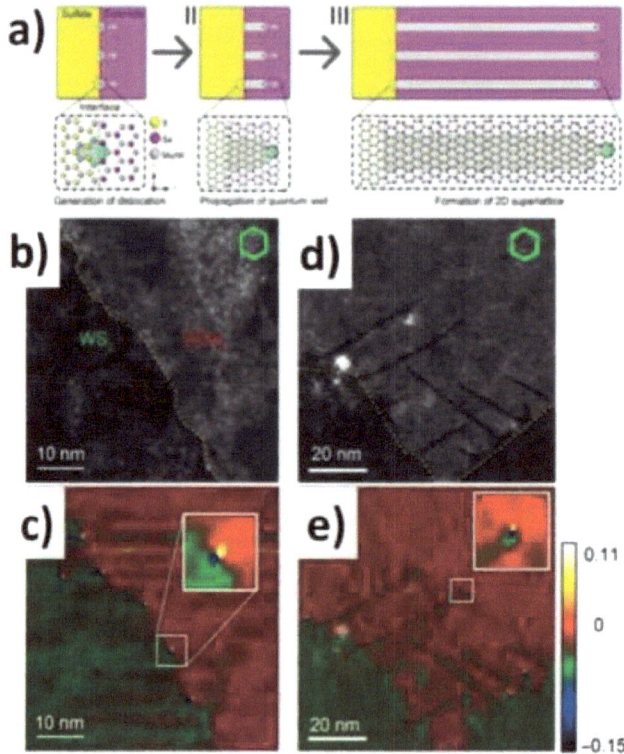

Fig. (1). Formation of periodic dislocation arrays and dislocation-driven growth of WS2 quantum wells at the WSe2/WS2 lateral interface. **a)** Schema showing (I) the formation of periodic dislocation array, (II) dislocation-driven growth of WS2 quantum wells and (III) formation of 2D quantum-well superlattice in the WSe2/WS2 lateral heterostructure. **b)** STEM-ADF image of a WSe2/WS2 lateral interface without the formation of WS2 quantum wells. The epitaxial interface is highlighted by the yellow dashed line. **c)** Corresponding strain distribution, overlaid onto the ADF image, shows the formation of periodic dislocation array at the heterointerface. **d)** STEM-ADF image of a WSe2/WS 2 lateral interface with the formation of WS2 quantum wells. The WS2 quantum wells are shown as darker stripes with the same width. **e)** Corresponding strain map, overlaid onto the ADF image, shows the presence of a dislocation core at the tip of each WS2 quantum well. Insets in (c) and (e) are magnified views of the strain maps at the highlighted dislocation cores [6].

Thus, based on modified and nano-patterned surfaces with the particular and controlled conductive properties, different optical circuits were fabricated for advanced applied quantum and photonics research. Accordingly, an experimental two-dimensional quantum walk of single electrons on a photonic chip [9] was reported. The quantum-enhanced power was related to the state of the quantum walks, expanded by enlarging the photon number and the dimensions of the evolution network with a diminished multiplicative loss of photons. In order to do that, 3D structures were accurately designed by laser irradiation with 49x49 nodes on a photonic chip, demonstrating the control of two-dimensional quantum walks using heralded single photons and single-photon level imaging. It was also possible to control ballistic evolution and variance of photons. From scalable monolithic circuit designs for an electro-optic device, including photon-pair regeneration, electro-optical path routing as well as voltage-controlled time delay of up to 12 ps on a single Ti:Li NbO^3 waveguide chip, manipulated photonic states were delivered by rotating polarization and control over single-qubit operations for potential applications to quantum computation and network [10].

Thus, from this brief discussion of a huge subject, it is possible to conclude that, by controlling the atomic level and sub-nm level, along with advanced laser excitation and election, quantum states and electronic conductions could be manipulated for applications in electronics and optoelectronics. Similar approaches leading to electromagnetic resonator applications such as wireless power transfer [11] and photonic conductions for light-fi applications [12] should also be mentioned.

CONCLUDING REMARKS

Optical and quantum circuits show a high impact on light and quantum technology developments from microelectronics, microprocessors and computer components to energy-harvesting devices such as solar cells. Although briefly discussed due to its ample scope, this topic showed how subwavelength phenomena could be sensed by new imaging modes, gaining a greater understanding of their effects for far-field developments.

REFERENCES

[1]   "Light management through guided mode resonances in thin film silicon solar cells", *J. of Nanophotonics,* vol. 8, pp. 1-14, 2014. 083995-1

[2]   B. Sain, R. Kaner, and Y. Prior, "Phase-controlled propagation of surface plasmons", *Light Sci. Appl.,* vol. 6, no. 10, p. e17072, 2017.
        [http://dx.doi.org/10.1038/lsa.2017.72] [PMID: 30167206]

[3]   N. Engheta, "Circuits with light at nanoscales: optical nanocircuits inspired by metamaterials", *Science,* vol. 317, no. 5845, pp. 1698-1702, 2007.
        [http://dx.doi.org/10.1126/science.1133268] [PMID: 17885123]

[4]   L. Zhang, X. Zhong, E. Pavlica, S. Li, A. Klekachev, G. Bratina, T. W. Ebbesen, E. Orgiu, and P. Samori, "A nanomesh scaffold for supramolecular nanowire optoelectronic devices", *Nature nanotech,* vol. 125, pp. 1-8, 2016.

[5]   P. Brown, K. Semeniuk, D. Wang, B. Monserrat, C. J. Pickard, and F. M. Grosche, "Strong coupling superconductivity in a quasiperiodic host guest structure", *Science Advances,* vol. 4, no. eaao4793, pp. 1-5, 2018.

[6]   W. Zhou, Y. Y. Zhang, J. Chen, D. Li, J. Zhou, Z. Liu, M. F. Chisholm, S. T. Pantelides, and K. Ping Loh, "Dislocation driven growth of two dimensional lateral quantum well superlattices", *Sci. Adv,* vol. 4, no. eaap9096, pp. 1-7, 2018.

[7] L. Fan, C. L. Zou, R. Cheng, X. Guo, X. Han, Z. Gong, S. Wang, and H. X. Tang, "Superconducting cavity electro-optics: A platform for coherent photon conversion between superconducting and photonics circuits", *Sci. Adv,* vol. 4, no. eaar4994, pp. 1-5, 2018.

[8] T. Zhong, J.M. Kindem, and J.G. Bartholomew, "Nanophotonicrare-earth quantum memory with optically controlled retrieval", *Science,* vol. 357, pp. 1392-1395, 2017.
[http://dx.doi.org/10.1126/science.aan5959] [PMID: 28860208]

[9] H. Tang, X. F. Lin, Z. Feng, J. Y. Chen, J. Gao, K. Sun, C. Y. Wang, P. C. Lai, X. Y. Xu, Y. Wang, L. F. Lai, X. Y. Xu, Y. Wang, L. F. Qiao, A. L. Yang, and X. M. Jin, "Experimental two dimensional quantum walk on a photonic chip", *Sci. Adv,* vol. 4, no. eaat3174, pp. 1-6, 2018.

[10] K. H. Luo, S. Brauer, C. Elgner, P. R. Sharapova, R. Ricken, T. Meier, H. Herrmann, and C. Silberhorn, "Nonlinear integrated quantum electro optic circuits", *Sci. Adv,* vol. 5, no. eaat1451, pp. 1-7, 2019.

[11] M. Song, P. Belov, and P. Kapitanova, "Wieless power transfer inspired by the modern trends in electromagnetics", *Appl. Phys. Rev.,* vol. 4, no. 021102, pp. 1-20, 2017.

[12] L. Yin, M.S. Islim, and H. Haas, "LiFi: Transforming Fibre into Wireless, Proc. SPIE 10128", *Broadband Access Communication Technologies XI,* vol. 1012802, pp. 1-9, 2017.

CHAPTER 10

Optosensors and Optrodes

Abstract: The use of optosensors and optrodes has shown high potential for targeted and controlled light emission delivery, as recorded from confined real sample volumes for different applications. In this way, we could stimulate the chromophores of biostructures incorporated in different tissues. It should be noted that different types of signaling could be recorded *in vivo*, such as electrophysiology, fluorescence signaling incorporating fluorescent reporters or an accurate excitation of fluorescent biostructures. In this chapter, different components for the fabrication of these types of reduced sized sensors are being reviewed, from the development of metamaterials to the modification of optical fibers, waveguides and use of light emitting devices (**LEDs**). The versatility of these sensors with respect to the design of injectable and implantable devices is also shown.

Keywords: Controlled light delivery, Electrophysiology tracking, Non-classical light recording, Optogenetics, Optrodes, Optosensors.

1. INTRODUCTION TO OPTODEVICES

Optosensors and different approaches range from in-flow approaches coupled with fluorescence spectroscopy by excitation with incorporated Standard Xenon Lamps [1] and by excitation and emission recording *via* optical fibers through reduced volume cells [2] for chemical sensing to the advanced design of optrodes based on optical fibers, micro-LEDs, conductive metamaterials and waveguides for high sensitive signal conduction. These incorporate lasers and highly sensitive detectors for *in vivo* optogenetics by targeted light delivery to *in vivo* tissues [3] (Fig. **1**).

Thus, with the appropriate light delivery, protein actuators could be activated, allowing the stimulation of the cell activity at different levels. For example, ion channels, ion pumps, as well as neurotransmitter tracking coupled with the electrophysiological recording by multimodal optical fiber optrodes (Fig. **2**).

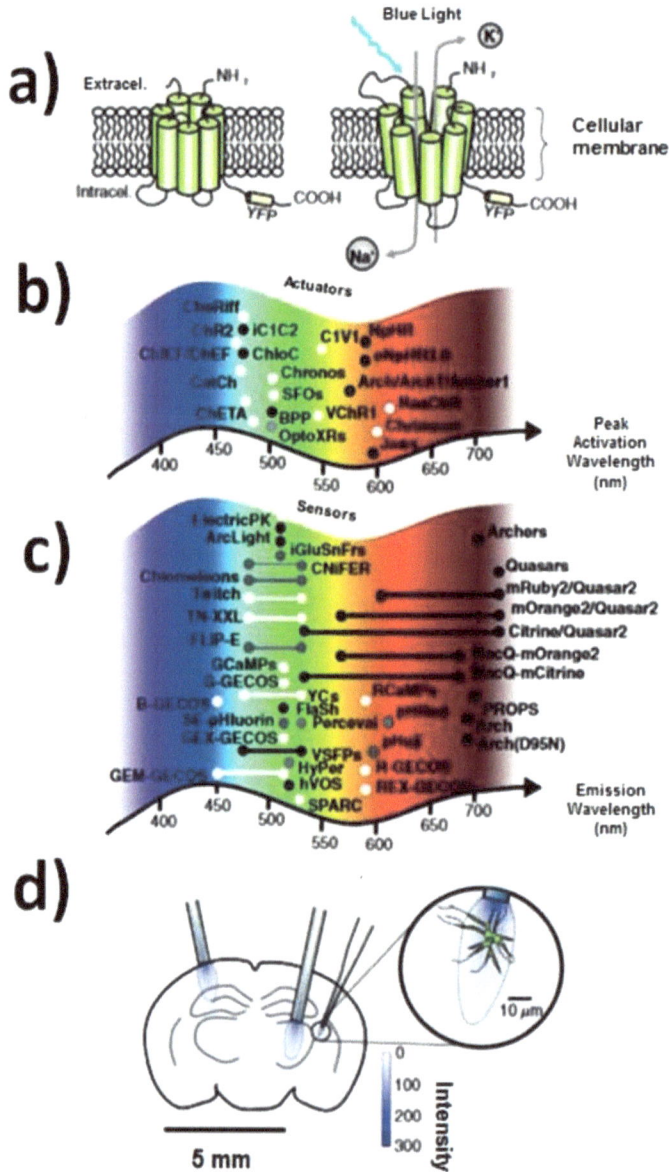

Fig. (1). Optogenetic tools and light tissue penetration. **a)** Schematic representation of a transmembrane channelrhodopsin protein in its closed (left) and opened (right) configurations following blue light illumination. **b)** and **c)** Schematic representation of the peak activation wavelength of the actuator (white)/silencing (black) proteins listed [16] and the fluorescent sensor proteins voltage (black), calcium (white), and other sensors (gray). Proteins for intracellular signaling control in panel b are represented in gray. **d)** Schematic representation of a coronal cross-section of a mouse brain illustrating the typical light penetrance achieved (distribution of irradiance, calculated using the equation in the Appendix) at 473 nm using a 200-μm diameter optical fiber (NA= 0.2) and a micro-optrode [3].

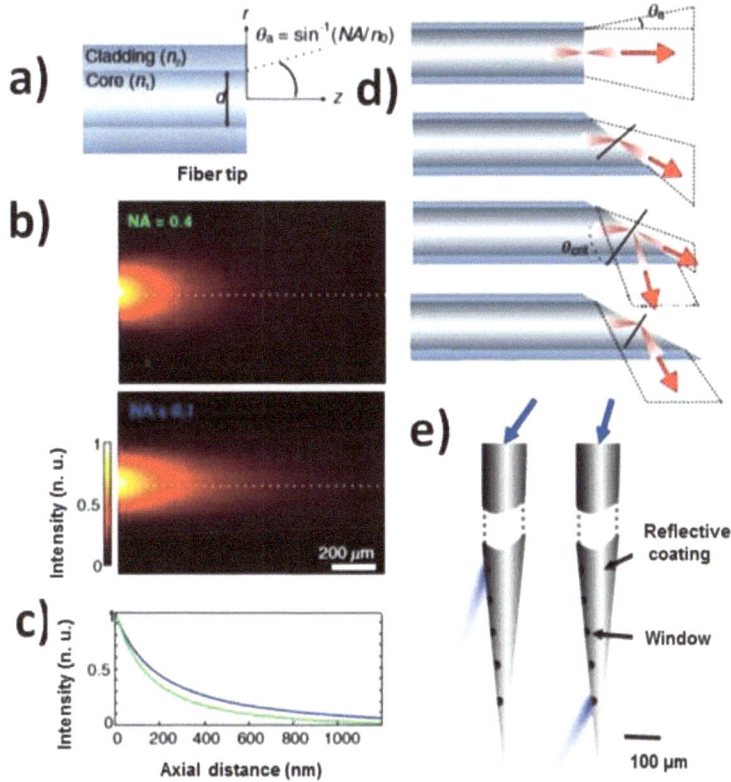

Fig. (2). Tissue irradiance profiles and strategies for controlled light delivery. **a)** Schematic representation of an optical fiber tip and the calculated irradiance profile. **b)** At its tip for NA=0.4 and NA=0.1, the diameter of the fiber core used in the calculation was 200 μm and values of absorption and scattering were chosen for a wavelength of 473nm. **c)** Axial normalized intensity profile at fiber center, corresponding to the dashed lines in (b). **d)** Different irradiance profiles obtained from different tip geometries. **e)** Flexible illumination location from a coated tapered fiber. Optical windows (≈5 μm wide) were made along the tapered shaft. Using different light input angles, different zones are illuminated [3].

2. DEVELOPMENT OF OPTOSENSORS AND OPTRODES

In order to develop portable micro- and nanodevices, the design, conformation and Implementation of optrodes should be discussed, for instance, cellular-scale optoelectronics applied to wireless optogenetics [4]. This advanced optrode was based on a multimodal optogenetic configuration used for freely moving animals. Hence, the microdevice between the nanoscale and below the millimeter was formed by an ultrathin multilayered device with the incorporation of electrode, micro-organic **LEDs**, temperature sensor and insertion needle, used for precision optical, thermal and electrophysiological sensors and actuators *via* wireless recording *in vivo*. This optrode microdevice showed high versatility due to its multimodal signal recording for brain sensing of free animals. However, these designs are still being developed in order to reduce their size for miniaturized optogenetic neural implants [5] based on advanced micro-technology with different light sources, including lasers, laser diodes and light-emitting diodes.

Then, we could discuss many variables related to signal transduction and approaches, which should be considered and improved for new metamaterial research [6]. For example, those based on fiber-waveguide coupling, on the incorporation of micro-LEDs; taking into account controlled wavelengths and light power of irradiance, coupling efficiency between the applied power of the source and the waveguide through different media and tissues, and as well as propagation efficiency and loss in waveguides.

Based on the design mentioned, different types of signaling could be recorded, such as fluorescence tracking from inter-neural connectivity by delivery of calcium and electrochemical neural activity sensing with potential applications in advanced electrophysiology, neuroscience and behavioral physiology [7]. It is therefore important to highlight the relevance of the development of different types of new materials with diverse properties, as discussed in previous sections. In this field, we can make reference, in particular, to the design of surface modifications for nanoscale sensor applications [8] with bioimplication in micro- and nanotechnologies for optical neural interfaces [9], where the surface chemistry of contact is particularly important due to biocompatibility and signal recording from the contact. The implication and applications of quantum phenomena of nano-sized materials are also important, in addition to their small size and high surface to volume ratios, potentially employed to investigate alternative strategies for building the next generation of optical neural interfaces and developing studies of tissues *in vivo*. In this way, the modification of waveguides and optical fiber grating for multimodal signal recording could be applied to the design of multimodal optrodes, for example, the development of metamaterial integration for fiber optics, leading to a dual effect of surface plasmon and classical waveguiding [10]. The metamaterial can be used as the core or cladding of a fiber, enabling waveguide through a subwavelength geometry. Other approaches linked to optical fiber, nanolasers and miniaturized optical tweezers for nanoparticle and molecule trapping are also worth noting, as in the use of hybrid nanoparticles as silica core gold shell nanoparticles for the fabrication of optical fiber long-period grating biosensor [11] for highly sensitive signal recording. These types of grating have improved fluorescence from a modified fiber optic biosensor with metallic nanoparticles [12] and fiber grating-assisted surface plasmon resonance for biochemical and electrochemical sensing [13]. Moreover, from a photonic nanojet generated by dielectric microlens bound to an optical fibre probe [14], three-dimensional manipulations were obtained for a single 85-nm fluorescent polystyrene nanoparticle as well as for a plasmid DNA molecule. In this respect, backscattering and fluorescent signals were detected with enhancement factors up to ~103 and ~30, respectively.

In summary, for the reduction of the size of optrodes towards miniaturized closed-loop optogenetic stimulation [15], their material composition is highly important due to their compact multi-component design. A closed-loop optogenetic stimulation system is formed basically by the implant of an electrode connected to the power source *via* the neural recorder with amplifier and bandpass filters, an LED connected to the optical fiber and the microcontroller and LED driver. Consequently, the appropriate tuning of each component of the materials and accurate control of the nanoscale should be applied.

CONCLUDING REMARKS

The control of light stimulation and recording along with the appropriate developments of the materials used have allowed their application in high-sensitive sensing from the *in vivo* region of the brain by a minimally invasive methodology to highly valuable information recording. Therefore, optosensing has a high potential for advanced medical diagnosis and new treatments.

REFERENCES

[1]   J. López-Flores, M.L. Fernández-De Córdova, and A. Molina-Díaz, "Multicommutated flow-through optosensors implemented with photochemically induced fluorescence: determination of flufenamic acid", *Anal. Biochem.,* vol. 361, no. 2, pp. 280-286, 2007.
      [http://dx.doi.org/10.1016/j.ab.2006.11.020] [PMID: 17188227]

[2]   J.F. Fernández-Sánchez, A. Segura-Carretero, J.M. Costa-Fernández, N. Bordel, R. Pereiro, C. Cruces-Blanco, A. Sanz-Medel, and A. Fernández-Gutiérrez, "Fluorescence optosensors based on different transducers for the determination of polycyclic aromatic hydrocarbons in water", *Anal. Bioanal. Chem.,* vol. 377, no. 4, pp. 614-623, 2003.
      [http://dx.doi.org/10.1007/s00216-003-2092-x] [PMID: 12845403]

[3]   S. Dufour, and Y. De Koninck, "Optrodes for combined optogenetics and electrophysiology in live animals", *Neurophotonics, 2, 3, 031205.,* pp. 1-14, 2015.

[4]   T.-i. Kim-M., "Injectable, cellular-scale optoelectronics with applications for wireless optogenetics", *Science,* vol. 340, no. 6129, pp. 211-216, 2013.
      [http://dx.doi.org/10.1126/science.1232437]

[5]   B. Fan, and W. Li, "Miniaturized optogenetic neural implants: a review,", *Lab on a Chip,* vol. 15, no. 19, pp. 3838-3855, 2015.

[6]   E. Iseri, and D. Kuzum, "Implantable optoelectronic probes for in vivo optogenetics", *J. Neural Eng.,* vol. 14, no. 3, 2017.031001
      [http://dx.doi.org/10.1088/1741-2552/aa60b3] [PMID: 28198703]

[7]   E.P. Kuleshova, "Optogenetics – New Potentials for Electrophysiology", *Neurosci. Behav. Physiol.,* vol. 49, no. 2, pp. 169-177, 2019.
      [http://dx.doi.org/10.1007/s11055-019-00711-5]

[8]   E. Reimhult, and F. Höök, "Design of surface modifications for nanoscale sensor applications", *Sensors (Basel),* vol. 15, no. 1, pp. 1635-1675, 2015.
      [http://dx.doi.org/10.3390/s150101635] [PMID: 25594599]

[9]   F. Pisanello, L. Sileo, and M. De Vittorio, "Micro- and nanotechnologies for optical neural interfaces",
        Front. Neurosci., vol. 10, no. 70, pp. 1-9, 2016.
        [http://dx.doi.org/10.3389/fnins.2016.00070]

[10]   E.J. Smith, Z. Liu, Y. Mei, and O.G. Schmidt, "Combined surface plasmon and classical waveguiding
        through metamaterial fiber design", *Nano Lett.,* vol. 10, no. 1, pp. 1-5, 2010.
        [http://dx.doi.org/10.1021/nl900550j] [PMID: 19368372]

[11]   L. Marques, F.U. Hernandez, S.W. James, S.P. Morgan, M. Clark, R.P. Tatam, and S. Korposh,
        "Highly sensitive optical fibre long period grating biosensor anchored with silica core gold shell
        nanoparticles", *Biosens. Bioelectron.,* vol. 75, pp. 222-231, 2016.
        [http://dx.doi.org/10.1016/j.bios.2015.08.046] [PMID: 26319165]

[12]   M-Y. Ng, and W-C. Liu, "Fluorescence enhancements of fiber-optic biosensor with metallic
        nanoparticles", *Opt. Express,* vol. 17, no. 7, pp. 5867-5878, 2009.
        [http://dx.doi.org/10.1364/OE.17.005867] [PMID: 19333356]

[13]   T. Guo, "Fiber grating-assisted surface plasmon resonance for biochemical and electrochemical
        sensing", *J. Lightwave Technol.,* vol. 35, no. 16, pp. 3323-3333, 2017.
        [http://dx.doi.org/10.1109/JLT.2016.2590879]

[14]   "2, H.-Bao Xin, H.-Xiang Lei, L.-L. Liu, Y.-Ze Li, Y. Zhang, B.-J. Li, Manipulation and detection of
        single nanoparticles and biomolecules by a photonic nanojet", *Light Sci. Appl.,* vol. 5, no. e16176, pp.
        1-9, 2016.

[15]   E.S. Edward, A.Z. Kouzani, and S.J. Tye, "Towards miniaturized closed-loop optogenetic stimulation
        devices", *J. Neural Eng.,* vol. 15, no. 2, 2018.021002
        [http://dx.doi.org/10.1088/1741-2552/aa7d62] [PMID: 29363618]

CHAPTER 11

Biophotonics at Single-Molecule Detection (SMD) Level

Abstract: Single-molecule detection (SMD) has shown to be a high-impact research field that could be developed based on nanoscale control with optical setups. In this way, different device and instrumental approaches could be implemented in biophotonic studies at SMD levels. For these reasons, varied designs of nanoplatforms, optical resonators, optical trapping, nano-patterned surfaces, and modified chemical surfaces are reviewed for SMD applications. In all these developments, signal transduction and enhancement led to the success of the targeted application. Therefore, we discuss here plasmonic [67] and enhanced plasmonic (EP) approaches, enhanced fluorescence signaling based on metal enhanced fluorescence (MEF) and plasmonic resonators, nanoantennas, and targeted molecular interactions by chemical modification of surfaces.

Keywords: Biophotonics, Molecular recognition, Nanophotonics, Optical resonator, Plasmonic nanoplatform, Single-molecule detection (SMD).

1. SINGLE-MOLECULE DETECTION

Within these fields, many approaches could be used to detect and track biomolecules and biostructures on the basis of different optical setups, from standard to advanced microscope techniques and advanced optical approaches as well, combining lens and high-power irradiancy lasers and high-sensitive detectors, depending on the spectroscopical properties studied. It is worth mentioning that a recent Nobel Prize-awarded development of super-resolved fluorescence microscopy [1] based on switched on/off of single molecular fluorescence [2, 3] was given in Chemistry, in 2014, to Germany and the USA. These levels of development and advanced resolution were carried out by controllable sources of single photons using optical pumping of single molecules in solids. Triggered single photons were produced at a high rate, whereas the probability of simultaneous emission of two photons is nearly zero-a useful property for **SMD** [4] and other applications, such asquantuminformation processing [5], quantum cryptography [6], and certain quantum computation problems [7]. Moreover, using transfected cells expressing modified, multi-fluorescent proteins with different emitters within a single diffraction limit, targeted regions were bonded.Thus, the contained information of the protein spatial organization was transferred to fluorescent emitter reporters linked, allowing, in this manner, a molecular resolution of the modified biostructure. Using this method, images of intracellular fluorescent proteins could be recorded with a nanometer resolution [8].

2. PLASMONIC NANOPLATFORMS FOR SMD

The ability to bring free-space electromagnetic optical radiations to the nanoscale with plasmonic nanostructures improved non-classical light for enhanced biosensing applications [9], as in ultra luminescent gold core-shell nanoparticles for bacteria labeling and single biostructure detection by laser fluorescence microscopy, in addition to potential applications, such as luminescent responsive nanoplatforms for molecular sensing. For the control of non-classical light emissions from controlled plasmon intensities based on the tuning of the nanoparticle sizes generated, different resolutions were achieved at the nanoscale in the design of advanced smart ultra-luminescent multifunctional nanoplatforms for biophotonic and nanomedicine applications [10].

Many single-molecule detection (**SMD**) approaches were designed with different plasmonic nanostructures with varied sizes, geometries, and materials, from individual to multiple nanoparticles in colloidal dispersion and nano-patterned surfaces. These nanoarchitectures were used as nanoplatforms for molecular recognition, trapping, and detection; many cases were based on imaging. Hence, optical detection of single molecules was achieved beyond the diffraction and diffusion limit [11].

In order to control the diffusion limit of the molecules, different intervals of concentrations were reported. Higher molecular concentrations were applied to overcome the diffusion limits; however, in real samples, low concentrations should be considered. In both cases, molecules should be recognized, captured or trapped, and detected based on the previous different enhanced phenomena discussed in the interactions with the high electromagnetic fields generated between confined resonant nanoantennas or by the use of tuned single nanoarchitectures.

In this way, we could report different approaches at lower concentrations. A case in point includes highly ordered modified surfaces with gold nano-patterned rods leading to enhanced fluorescence imaging based on **MEF**, which allowed **SMD** of the fluorescent reporter evaluated at low concentrations [12] (Fig. **1**).

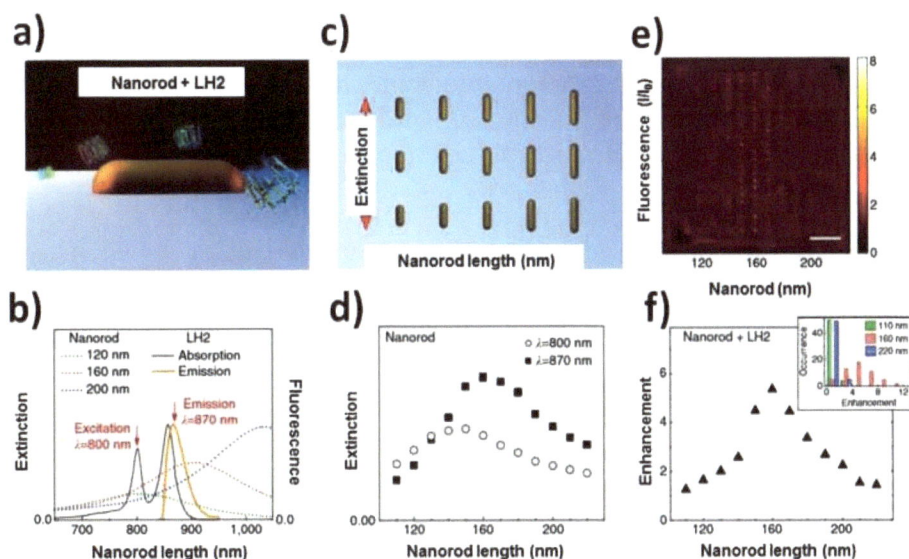

Fig. (1). Coupling LH2 to a gold nanoantenna in an ensemble measurement at low concentration. **a)** Schematic presentation of a gold NR with an LH2 complex located in the antenna hot spot. **b)** Absorption and emission spectra of LH2 in solution and extinction spectra of L=120, 160 and 200nm NRs. The extinction spectra were measured with the polarization of the incident light parallel to the long antenna axis. **c)** Schematic presentation of the NR array with increasing antenna length. The polarization of the excitation light is parallel to the NRs. **d)** Extinction of the antennas at the excitation (l=800nm) and emission (l=870nm) wavelength as a function of antenna length. **e)** Confocal fluorescence image of LH2 in PVA spin-coated over NRs with length increasing from L=110–220nm. The intensity is normalized to the unenhanced emission coming from B800 LH2s in our diffraction limited focus. Scale bar, 10mm. **f)** Average fluorescence enhancement. The maximal enhancement is reached for L=160nm Au NRs. Inset: histogram of the enhancement for 54 Au NRs of L=110, 160 and 220nm [12].

Moreover, by transmission electron microscopy focused on single silver nanocubes, the mapping of the enhanced quantum efficiency of the molecular dipole emitters was afforded based on their position on the Nano-surfaces at low concentration intervals. These assays were in the order of femtomolar (10^{-15}) or attomolar (10^{-18}) intervals where a diffusion limitation took place from the bulk to the nanoplatform , adding extra time to the detection of the molecular event.

Approaches at higher concentration intervals based on different plasmonic phenomena could be mentioned as well. For example, antenna-in-box platforms for enhanced single-molecule analysis were reported by enhanced fluorescence from enhanced plasmonic interactions [13].

Moreover, individual gold nanoparticles were also developed for an enhanced single molecule by fluorescence co rrelation spectroscopy, showing temporal fluctuations of the emissions in the presence and absence of fluorescent reporters at micromolar concentration [14]. From these assays, the 0.5 fL confocal detection volume (diffraction-limited) contained about 3000 molecules at the targeted concentration of fluorescent molecules of 10 μ M, while only a few molecules were expected to be in the sub-attoliter near-field volume around the nanoparticle that generated variation in the emission signal recorded.

At higher concentrated fluorescent reporter concentrations such as 25 μM, self-assembled DNA origami-based optical nanoantennas were developed. This DNA based nanostructure showed improved interparticle distance accompanied by an optimized quantum-yield that permitted an enhancement factor of more than 5000-fold fluorescence [15].

In addition, in other approaches based on resonant cavities, single-molecule optomechanical detection was performed within "picocavity dimensions in cryogenic conditions [16]. In this way, the diffraction limit was reached and allowed light trapping within volumes of 30 cubic nanometers and below 1 cubic nanometer ("picocavities"), enabling optical experiments on the atomic scale.

These atomic features were dynamically formed and disassembled by laser irradiation. Following this extreme optical confinement approach, yields of factors of 106 enhancement of optomechanical coupling were recorded between the picocavity field and vibrations of individual molecular bonds. Hence, a nonlinear quantum optical system was studied for single-molecule level detection.

3. SUPRAMOLECULAR, DNA-BASED AND OTHER SMD APPROACHES

The molecular, nanostructured, and laser-based approaches of **SMD** previously mentioned were based on enhanced strategies by different phenomena applications. Yet, a challenge is still being posed in relation to molecular recognition in real samples, low concentrations, labeling, and diffusional limitations, *etc.*, requiring developments of new **SMD** methodologies based on the different phenomena discussed, in terms of the application and targeted molecules as well as of the implementation of other approaches of **SMD** and proofs of concepts.

Regarding these new proofs of concepts and other **SMD** strategies already developed as well as currently in progress, we can refer to the incorporation of supramolecular systems, such as cyclodextrins as a supramolecular host-guest complex formation strategy, which showed a decrease in and prevention of static quenching of conjugated polymer fluorescence at the single-molecule level [17].

Moreover, the use of functional bio-interactions as enzymatic systems allowed developing enzyme-linked immunosorbent assay that detected serum proteins at subfemtomolar concentrations [18] at **SMD** level. In this way, an approach for simultaneously detecting hundreds to thousands of individual protein molecules was reported, enabling the detection of very low concentrations of proteins. Proteins were captured on microscopic beads and labeled with an enzyme. Each bead had either one or zero enzyme-labeled proteins. By isolating these beads in arrays of 50-femtoliter reaction chambers, it achieved single protein detections by fluorescence imaging.

Note that high-impact research was developed for DNA detection and amplification, based on different optical approaches and controlled DNA grafting of surfaces [19]. For single-molecule sequencing, for example, we may refer to sequencing and tracking of individual nucleotides based on a templated DNA exposed to a solution containing DNA polymerase and a fluorescent nucleotide. If a nucleotide were incorporated, it would be achieved by a complementary strand of the template. Thus, the fluorescence would be read using a total internal reflection fluorescence (TIRF)-based Helioscope, recording the positions where the DNA strand had incorporated a fluorescent nucleotide from the solution [20]. It should also be noted that real-time DNA sequencing from single polymerase molecules [21] enabled tracking of single nucleotide incorporation in real-time by fluorescence imaging. The level of developments achieved in single-molecule dynamic detection of chemical reactions [22] based on an electrochemical device is also worth noting.

4. OPTICAL TWEEZERS

First of all, it should be noted that optical tweezers to control nanoparticles to microparticles based on commercially advanced instrumentations [23] and new setups were developed. Such as for example, the use of two optical microscopes placed on the axial and lateral positions, to focus on small volumes for particles targeting [24], based on scattering forces from both incident beams at the sides.

Accordingly, the optical manipulation of particles led to molecular detection over their surfaces based on spectroscopical, physical, and chemistry modifications recorded by different detection techniques. For instance, optical tweezers showed a high sensitive single DNA strand detection based on single-molecule force spectroscopy for studies linked to mechanisms of DNA binding determined by optical tweezers on trapped microparticles (Fig. **2**) [25]. Therefore, a streptavidin-coated polystyrene bead with a diameter of 5 µm was introduced into the solution and ultimately held in the trap, while another was attached to a micropipette tip.

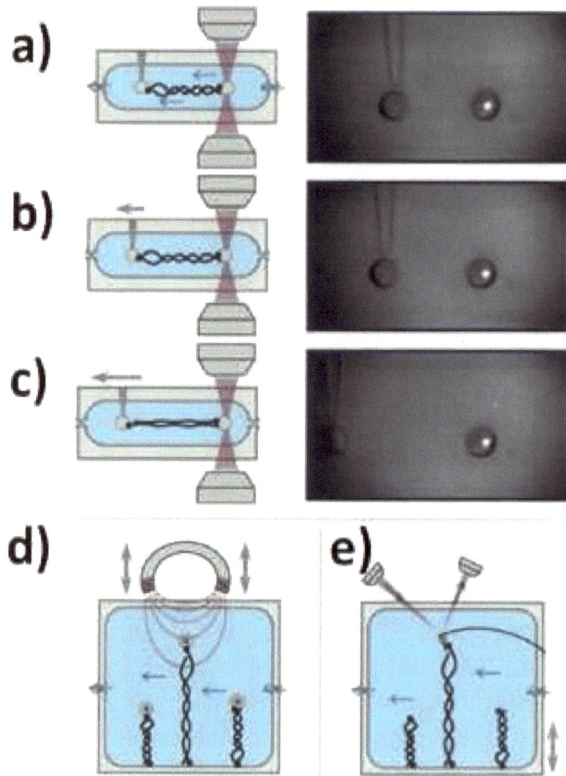

Fig. (2). Force spectroscopy of single molecules. **a)** In this optical tweezer scheme, the vertical counter-propagating beams are focused on the right, within the grey flow cell. A streptavidin-coated polystyrene bead (open circle) is held in the trap formed by the beams, while another is attached to the glass micropipette tip on the left. Biotinylated DNA molecules are ''caught'' and suspended between the two beads. The double helix may be stretched. **b)** and melted; **c)** in the absence and presence of binding drugs or proteins. The pictures to the right show the beads (5 m diameter), the laser focus (1 m) and the DNA (not visible) at various extensions of the cell. The change in position of the cell within the trap determines the applied force. **d)** Magnetic tweezers extend DNA tethered between a magnetic bead and a streptavidin-coated cover slip. Increasing the strength of the magnetic field increases the applied force. **e)** In force microscopy experiments, DNA is stretched between a cover slip and a cantilever. As the cell is moved, the deflection of a laser by the cantilever records the force on the double helix [25].

A solution containing phage lambda DNA (48,500 base pairs, biotin labeled on each 30 terminus) or similar DNA was introduced into the cell, allowing DNA attachment between the beads. The DNA solution consisted of 10 mM Hepes, pH 7.5, and Na^+ ions at a controlled concentration (typically 100 mM). The cell, mounted on a piezoelectric stage, may be moved with nanometer precision, causing the DNA to stretch between the two beads. As the force upon the DNA increased, the bead in the optical trap was displaced, generating a beam deflection that may be determined on the lateral effect detectors. In this manner, forces up to 300 pN with a resolution of 1 pN were determined. Moreover, high sensitivity was found against specific ligands to the double strands such as nuclearproteins and non-specific interactions, molecular intercalants, and media changes. Thus, it was shown how important information on the dynamics of DNA at the **SMD** level could be recorded from microparticle platform appropriately tuned.

In addition, other strategies could be applied for **SMD** developments. For instance, long-range optical trapping and binding of microparticles in hollow-core photonic crystal fibers [26] were developed. In this manner, molecular events were detected and tracked on single particle surfaces by different optical detection systems. So, the importance of the application of optical tweezers for **SMD** based on tracking of appropriate chemical modified particle platforms could be observed from different approaches.

CONCLUDING REMARKS

The detection of biomolecules at the SMD level still poses a major challenge due to which it should be recorded from the bulk targeted molecular signaling. In this manner, the interaction of the single molecule should be specific and accompanied by enhanced signal transduction in order to be detected. For these reasons, the control of the nanoscale allowed the use of nanoplatforms for the deposition of a varied number of molecules by adjusting the molecular concentrations. However, even if these approaches were used with small aliquots in confined volumes,it should overcome the interactions and matrix effects with interferent analytes in real samples. Additionally, for biophotonic measurements in vivo, additional challenges should be met for the incorporation of nanodevices and microdevices into the tissues by injection, for the implementation of implantable approaches, and for a controlled light delivery using modified optical fibers as well.

REFERENCES

[1]   E. Betzig, S.W. Hell, and W.E. Moerner, "The Nobel Prize in Chemistry 2014, for the development of super-resolved fluorescence microscopy", *Press Release from the Royal Swedish Academy of Sciences,* 2014.

[2]   S.W. Hell, and J. Wichmann, "Breaking the diffraction resolution limit by stimulated emission: stimulated-emission-depletion fluorescence microscopy", *Opt. Lett.,* vol. 19, no. 11, pp. 780-782, 1994.
[http://dx.doi.org/10.1364/OL.19.000780] [PMID: 19844443]

[3]   S.W. Hell, "Nanoscopy with Focused Light (Nobel Lecture)", *Angew. Chem. Int. Ed. Engl.,* vol. 54, no. 28, pp. 8054-8066, 2015.
[http://dx.doi.org/10.1002/anie.201504181] [PMID: 26088439]

[4]   B. Lounis, and W.E. Moerner, "Single photons on demand from a single molecule at room temperature", *Nature,* vol. 407, no. 6803, pp. 491-493, 2000.
[http://dx.doi.org/10.1038/35035032] [PMID: 11028995]

[5]   "Special issue on quantum information", *Phys. World,* vol. 11, no. 3, 1998.

[6]   C.H. Bennett, G. Brassard, and A.K. Ekert, "Quantum cryptography", *Sci. Am.,* vol. 267, no. 4, pp. 50-57, 1992.
       [http://dx.doi.org/10.1038/scientificamerican1092-50]

[7]   Q.A. Turchette, C.J. Hood, W. Lange, H. Mabuchi, and H.J. Kimble, "Measurement of conditional phase shifts for quantum logic", *Phys. Rev. Lett.,* vol. 75, no. 25, pp. 4710-4713, 1995.
       [http://dx.doi.org/10.1103/PhysRevLett.75.4710] [PMID: 10059978]

[8]   E. Betzig, G.H. Patterson, R. Sougrat, O. Wolf Lindwasser, and J.S. Scott Olenych, "Imaging intracellular fluorescent proteins at nanometer resolution", *Science,* vol. 313, no. 57931, pp. 642-1645, 2006.

[9]   J. Guo, J. R. Hendrickson, and T. S. Luk, "Special section guest editorial: nanoplasmonics for biosensing and enhanced light-matter interaction", *J. Nanophoton,* vol. 12,1, no. 012501, pp. 1-2, 2017.

[10]   C. Salinas, and G. Bracamonte, "Design of advanced smart ultraluminescent multifunctional nanoplatforms for biophotonics and nanomedicine applications, frontiers in drug", *Chemistry and Clinical Research,* vol. 1, no. 1, pp. 1-8, 2018.

[11]   F. Karim, T. B. Smith, and C. Zhao, "Review of optical detection of single molecules beyond the diffraction and diffusion limit using plasmonic nanostructures", *J. Nanophotonics,* vol. 12,1, no. 012504, pp. 1-15, 2017.

[12]   E. Wientjes, J. Renger, A.G. Curto, R. Cogdell, and N.F. van Hulst, "Strong antenna-enhanced fluorescence of a single light-harvesting complex shows photon antibunching", *Nat. Commun.,* vol. 5, p. 4236, 2014.
       [http://dx.doi.org/10.1038/ncomms5236] [PMID: 24953833]

[13]   D. Punj, M. Mivelle, S.B. Moparthi, T.S. van Zanten, H. Rigneault, N.F. van Hulst, M.F. García-Parajó, and J. Wenger, "A plasmonic 'antenna-in-box' platform for enhanced single-molecule analysis at micromolar concentrations", *Nat. Nanotechnol.,* vol. 8, no. 7, pp. 512-516, 2013.
       [http://dx.doi.org/10.1038/nnano.2013.98] [PMID: 23748196]

[14]   D. Punj, J. de Torres, H. Rigneault, and J. Wenger, "Gold nanoparticles for enhanced single molecule fluorescence analysis at micromolar concentration", *Opt. Express,* vol. 21, no. 22, pp. 27338-27343, 2013.
       [http://dx.doi.org/10.1364/OE.21.027338] [PMID: 24216956]

[15]   A. Puchkova, C. Vietz, E. Pibiri, B. Wünsch, M. Sanz Paz, G.P. Acuna, and P. Tinnefeld, "DNA Origami Nanoantennas with over 5000-fold Fluorescence Enhancement and Single-Molecule Detection at 25 μM", *Nano Lett.,* vol. 15, no. 12, pp. 8354-8359, 2015.
       [http://dx.doi.org/10.1021/acs.nanolett.5b04045] [PMID: 26523768]

[16]   F. Benz, M.K. Schmidt, A. Dreismann, R. Chikkaraddy, Y. Zhang, A. Demetriadou, C. Carnegie, H. Ohadi, B. de Nijs, R. Esteban, J. Aizpurua, and J.J. Baumberg, "Single-molecule optomechanics in "picocavities"", *Science,* vol. 354, no. 6313, pp. 726-729, 2016.
       [http://dx.doi.org/10.1126/science.aah5243] [PMID: 27846600]

[17]   D. Thomsson, R. Camacho, Y. Tian, D. Yadav, G. Sforazzini, H.L. Anderson, and I.G. Scheblykin, "Cyclodextrin insulation prevents static quenching of conjugated polymer fluorescence at the single molecule level", *Small,* vol. 9, no. 15, pp. 2619-2627, 2013.
       [http://dx.doi.org/10.1002/smll.201203272] [PMID: 23463732]

[18]   D.M. Rissin, C.W. Kan, T.G. Campbell, S.C. Howes, D.R. Fournier, L. Song, T. Piech, P.P. Patel, L. Chang, A.J. Rivnak, E.P. Ferrell, J.D. Randall, G.K. Provuncher, D.R. Walt, and D.C. Duffy, "Single-molecule enzyme-linked immunosorbent assay detects serum proteins at subfemtomolar concentrations", *Nat. Biotechnol.,* vol. 28, no. 6, pp. 595-599, 2010.
       [http://dx.doi.org/10.1038/nbt.1641] [PMID: 20495550]

[19]   D.R. Walt, "Optical methods for single molecule detection and analysis", *Anal. Chem.,* vol. 85, no. 3,

pp. 1258-1263, 2013.
[http://dx.doi.org/10.1021/ac3027178] [PMID: 23215010]

[20]   I. Braslavsky, B. Hebert, E. Kartalov, and S.R. Quake, "Sequence information can be obtained from single DNA molecules", *Proc. Natl. Acad. Sci. USA,* vol. 100, no. 7, pp. 3960-3964, 2003.
[http://dx.doi.org/10.1073/pnas.0230489100] [PMID: 12651960]

[21]   J. Eid, A. Fehr, J. Gray, K. Luong, J. Lyle, G. Otto, P. Peluso, D. Rank, P. Baybayan, B. Bettman, A. Bibillo, K. Bjornson, B. Chaudhuri, F. Christians, R. Cicero, S. Clark, R. Dalal, A. Dewinter, J. Dixon, M. Foquet, A. Gaertner, P. Hardenbol, C. Heiner, K. Hester, D. Holden, G. Kearns, X. Kong, R. Kuse, Y. Lacroix, S. Lin, P. Lundquist, C. Ma, P. Marks, M. Maxham, D. Murphy, I. Park, T. Pham, M. Phillips, J. Roy, R. Sebra, G. Shen, J. Sorenson, A. Tomaney, K. Travers, M. Trulson, J. Vieceli, J. Wegener, D. Wu, A. Yang, D. Zaccarin, P. Zhao, F. Zhong, J. Korlach, and S. Turner, "Real-time DNA sequencing from single polymerase molecules", *Science,* vol. 323, no. 5910, pp. 133-138, 2009.
[http://dx.doi.org/10.1126/science.1162986] [PMID: 19023044]

[22]   J. Guan, C. Jia, Y. Li, Z. Liu, J. Wang, Z. Yang, C. Gu, D. Su, K. N. Houk, D. Zhang, and X. Guo, "Direct single molecule dynamic detection of chemical reactions", *Sci. Adv,* vol. 4, no. eaar2177, pp. 1-8, 2018.

[23]   J. N. A. Mathews, "Commercial optical traps emerge from biophysics labs", *Physics Today,* vol. 62,2, no. 26, pp. 26-27, 2009.

[24]   P. Zemánek, A. Jonás, L. Srámek, and M. Liska, "Optical trapping of nanoparticles and microparticles by a Gaussian standing wave", *Opt. Lett.,* vol. 24, no. 21, pp. 1448-1450, 1999.
[http://dx.doi.org/10.1364/OL.24.001448] [PMID: 18079828]

[25]   M.J. McCauley, and M.C. Williams, "Mechanisms of DNA binding determined in optical tweezers experiments", *Biopolymers,* vol. 85, no. 2, pp. 154-168, 2007.
[http://dx.doi.org/10.1002/bip.20622] [PMID: 17080421]

[26]   D.S. Bykov, S. Xie, R. Zeltner, A. Machnev, G.K.L. Wong, T.G. Euser, and P.S.J. Russell, "Long-range optical trapping and binding of microparticles in hollow-core photonic crystal fibre", *Light Sci. Appl.,* vol. 7, no. 22, p. 22, 2018.
[http://dx.doi.org/10.1038/s41377-018-0015-z] [PMID: 30839617]

CHAPTER 12

Miniaturized Microscopes

Abstract: Recent developments in miniaturized instrumentation resulted in the design and fabrication of miniaturized microscopes with high versatility and application in neurophotonics, using portable miniaturized microscopes and even reduced-size wireless microscopes incorporated into rodent skulls, allowing different types of signal tracking and highly valuable information recording from neuro-emitters, ion channel gates, neuron interactions and other types of brain cells and that based on microscopy imaging *in vivo*. Here, we discuss the versatility and state-of-the-art technology of these miniaturized instrumentations.

Keywords: Endoscope, Miniaturized instrumentation, Miniaturized microscope, Neuroimaging, Portable wireless microscope.

1. INTRODUCTION

The large development trajectory and high impact on research and industry by the use of different microscopy techniques in numerous scientific areas led to the development of new microscopes, techniques, and methodologies. Then, with the arrival of the miniaturization of instruments, new types of imaging systems were developed by a combination of lasers, LEDs, optical fibers, and optics.

2. VERSATILITY AND APPLICATIONS OF MINIATURIZED INSTRUMENTATION

In vivo biosensing through optical fiber by imaging contributed to the design and application of compact instrumentations, such as endoscopes, for *in vivo* calcium imaging in freely behaving mice [1]. However, due to the need for higher resolution from multimodal approaches, developments of compact imaging instrumentation were accompanied by the development of miniaturized instrumentation. In neuroscience, particularly, data acquisition from inter-cell communication, neurotransmitter tracking, and biological event tracking *in vivo* is of high impact in different research fields. Similarly, detection of early cancer cells and chemical modifications within cells motivated new imaging techniques towards miniaturized imaging systems [2].

In this manner, the application of mini scopes and miniaturized microscopes has allowed transcending the limitations of resolution of single-neuron analysis in order to understand complex relations between cell signaling and behavior based on *in vivo* studies [3].

Moreover, the mini-microscopes developed for research have led to the design of commercial instrumentation currently in progress. Miniaturization went hand in hand with the incorporation of other imaging modes and techniques such as the integration of miniaturized fluorescence microscopy [4]. Hence, fluorescence imaging was applied through head-mounted microscopes in freely behaving animals, turning into a standard method to study neural circuit function.

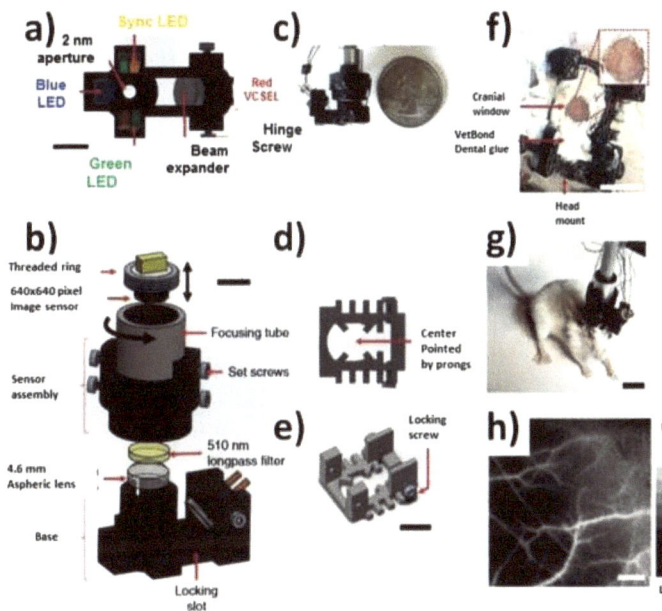

Fig. (1). Miniature plug-and-play design with three optical contrast mechanisms. **a)** A bottom view of the microscope base unit. Excitation for green fluorescent imaging is provided by a blue LED, while HbT imaging is carried out with a pair of green LEDs. A red laser diode, in conjunction with a beam expander and hinge screws, [commas] facilitates dHb and LSC imaging. A separate pair of orange (sync) LEDs is used for synchronizing with external instruments (*e.g.*, an EEG system). The FoV lies directly below the aperture. **b)** The sensor unit of the microscope shown along the base consists of a 4.6mm focal length lens, a 510nm long-pass filter to block blue fluorescence excitation light, a focusing tube, and an image sensor. **c)** The complete microscope assembly is shown with a U.S. quarter coin next to it for scale. **d), e)** Bottom and side views of the head mount, respectively. The head mount is surgically implanted on the rodent's skull and enables firm attachment of the microscope *via* a pair of locking screws. The pronged structure at the base of the head mount facilitates centering on the FoV. **f)** Head mount attached to a mouse skull with the inset showing the cranial window for optical access to the brain. **g)** A freely moving mouse with the microscope. **h)** A grayscale CBF map acquired with the microscope from an awake mouse using LSC imaging. The microscope housing was rapidly prototyped and 3D printed, allowing a high degree of customization. Scale bar indicates 5mm in (a), (b), and (f), 1cm in g, and 500μm in (h). Also, see Supplementary Figs. **1, 2** and **3**.

In addition, a growing open source community of researchers recently developed Flexible and affordable wide-field miniature microscopes, including the UCLA (University of California in Los Angeles) miniscope [5]. This miniscope has contributed to advancedresearch into *in vivo* neural inter-relationships linked to distinct contextual memories encoded close in time. Yet, such studies also need to monitor the behavior in order to correlate behavior and neuronal activity and also manipulate neuronal activity to determine causality in neuronal circuitry. Due to the major implications involved, interest in such research has grown in areas ranging from cell biology to social behaviour.

Consequently, this imaging methodology, together with fluorescent sensors freely behaving in animals, was selected as the method of the year 2018 [6]. This miniaturized optical instrumentation also showed the same versatilities in advanced microscopy, as in fast high-resolution miniature two-photon microscopy for brain imaging in freely behaving mice [7] and in multi-contrast microscopy for functional imaging in freely behaving animals [8] (Fig. **1**). This technology was even developed for an open-source and wireless system [9].

CONCLUDING REMARKS

Miniaturized microscopy, based on reduced-size optics, light-emitting devices (**LEDs**), optical fibers, and other technological parts, such as cameras and wireless antennas, has allowed neuroimaging *in vivo*. These instrumental developments permitted high precision research studies, such as on free rodents for *in vivo* data recording of neuro-interactions accompanied by correlations with their behavior.

REFERENCES

[1]   A.D. Jacob, A.I. Ramsaran, A.J. Mocle, L.M. Tran, C. Yan, P.W. Frankland, and S.A. Josselyn, "A compact head-mounted endoscope for in vivo calcium imaging in freely behaving mice", *Curr. Protoc. Neurosci.,* vol. 84, no. 1, 2018.e51
[http://dx.doi.org/10.1002/cpns.51] [PMID: 29944206]

[2]   M.R. Descour, A.H.O. Kärkkäinen, J.D. Rogers, C. Liang, R.S. Weinstein, J.T. Rantala, B. Kilic, E. Madenci, R.R. Richards-Kortum, E.V. Anslyn, R.D. Dupuis, R.J. Schul, C.G. Willison, and C.P. Tigges, "Toward the development of miniaturized imaging systems for detection of pre-cancer", *IEEE J. Quantum Electron.,* vol. 38, no. 2, pp. 122-130, 2002.
[http://dx.doi.org/10.1109/3.980264]

[3]   D. Aharoni, B.S. Khakh, A.J. Silva, and P. Golshani, "All the light that we can see: a new era in miniaturized microscopy", *Nat. Methods,* vol. 16, no. 1, pp. 11-13, 2019.
[http://dx.doi.org/10.1038/s41592-018-0266-x] [PMID: 30573833]

[4]   K.K. Ghosh, L.D. Burns, E.D. Cocker, A. Nimmerjahn, Y. Ziv, A.E. Gamal, and M.J. Schnitzer, "Miniaturized integration of a fluorescence microscope", *Nat. Methods,* vol. 8, no. 10, pp. 871-878, 2011.
[http://dx.doi.org/10.1038/nmeth.1694] [PMID: 21909102]

[5]   D. J. Cail, D. Aharoni, T. Shuman, J. Shobe, J. Biane, W. Song, B. Wei, M. Veshkini, M. La-Vul, J. Lou, S. Flores, I. Kim, Y. Sano, M. Zhou, K. Baumgaertel, A. Lavi, M. Kamata, M. Tuszynski, M. Mayford, P. Golshani, and A. J. Silva, "A shared neural ensemble links distinct contextual memories encoded close in time", *Nature,* vol. 534, pp. 115-131, 2016.

[6]   "Method of the year 2018: imaging in freely behaving animals, nature communications", *Editorial,* vol. 16, p. 1, 2019.

[7]   W. Zong, R. Wu, M. Li, Y. Hu, Y. Li, J. Li, H. Rong, H. Wu, Y. Xu, Y. Lu, H. Jia, M. Fan, Z. Zhou, Y. Zhang, A. Wang, L. Chen, and H. Cheng, "Fast high-resolution miniature two-photon microscopy for brain imaging in freely behaving mice", *Nat. Methods,* vol. 14, no. 7, pp. 713-719, 2017. [http://dx.doi.org/10.1038/nmeth.4305] [PMID: 28553965]

[8]   J. Senarathna, H. Yu, C. Deng, A.L. Zou, J.B. Issa, D.H. Hadjiabadi, S. Gil, Q. Wang, B.M. Tyler, N.V. Thakor, and A.P. Pathak, "A miniature multi-contrast microscope for functional imaging in freely behaving animals", *Nat. Commun.,* vol. 10, no. 1, p. 99, 2019. [http://dx.doi.org/10.1038/s41467-018-07926-z] [PMID: 30626878]

[9]   W. A. Liberti, L. Nathan Perkins, D. P. Leman, and T. J. Gardner, "An open source, wireless capable miniature microscope system", *J Neural Eng,* vol. 14, no. 4, pp. 1-17.

Frontiers in Nano-and Micro-device Design, 2021, 111-121   111

CHAPTER 13

Neurophotonics

Abstract: Neurophotonics has aroused considerable interest over the last years due to the information recorded from in-vivo animals by applying light-controlled excitation and emission recording. In this section, we discuss the main labelling techniques, molecular and ion reporters and optical approaches available. Recent studies also show the application of optosensor, implantable microdevices, and knowledge from neurophotonics to the design of microdevices and circuits that mimics neuro-interactions.

Keywords: Labelling technique, Neuro-electrophysiology, Neuroimaging, Neurophotonics, Neurotransmitter tracking, Photonics.

1. INTRODUCTION

Neurophotonics studies light from different sources with neurons and brain cells in order to better understand their inter-connection, functionality, neuro-biological event changes and different healthy-unhealthy states of the brain. From early neuroscience to neurophotonic studies based on advanced optical techniques, significant insights have been provided at the macro-, meso-, micro- and nano-scale.

In this brief section, it was described the importance of this research field accompanied with a discussion of the main themes related. The optical developments for brain imaging and analysis of confined brain volumes by laser irradiation and miniaturization of instrumentation.

Considering the complexity of the brain function?, not all electromagnetic field wavelengths could be applied to excite the samples. In view of this, we will refer to spectroscopical techniques and advanced optical setups within the infrared interval [1], fluorescence [2], fluorescence microscopy [3], magnetic resonance [4], acoustic, photoacoustic wavelengths [5], scattered light-based techniques [6] and multimodal modes [7]. Thus, from the spectroscopical techniques indicated, the information could be recorded from the brain and single-cell signaling to image recording.

A. Guillermo Bracamonte

2. LABELLING TECHNIQUES

It is then possible to analyze samples of rodent and human post-mortem brain tissues with *in vivo* imaging. In this manner, this type of study permitted real-time data collection. For brain imaging of small animals such as rodents, retrograde labeling [8] *via* targeted viral infection at their terminal neuro-structures has allowed correlating their projections and inter-connections [9]. These labelled tissues were analyzed from post-mortem by sectioning the brain in multiple slides to obtain rodent brain imaging of the whole organ and extract single neurons [10].

Traditional staining methods based on immunochemistry for neurobiology [11] have also allowed specific neuro-labelling of different parts of neuro-structures. Additionally, fluorescent molecular probes have been used in protein recognition [12], for instance, in tyrosine hydroxylase identification, detection and quantification, enabling its topological organization and phenotypic plasticity study [13].

A further well-known labelling technique for gene expression of cells and neurons comprises fluorescent *in situ* hybridization (FISH), demonstrating precise localization of a targeted segment of nucleic acid in a histologic section. The underlying basis of FISH was by the application of a complementary strand of nucleic acids covalently labelled with fluorescent reporters for detection of the targeted strand after hybridization based on the emission signal tracking of the incorporated reporter molecule. By this manner, it was allowed the localization of specific DNA and RNA strands [14].

In addition, the application of multimodal nanoparticles for neuro-labelling, such as bi-functional magneto-fluorescent contrast agents is also found in the literature [15]. Then, although such methods enhanced resolution and specificity in different parts of neurons, as compared to non-invasive imaging techniques such as magnetic resonance imaging (MRI), and outperformed light microscopy in field of view and depth of imaging, they did not offer cellular resolution and specificity, in addition to low signal-to-noise ratio and low temporal resolution.

In view of this, according to the different labelling procedures discussed, it is possible to target specific brain regions, cell and neuron membranes in order to generate bioimaging. From the different imaging modes developed a high level of data recording for biostructure characterization and biological event tracking.

3. FROM BASIC RESEARCH TO ADVANCED METHODOLOGIES FOR BRAIN IMAGING

Controlled multi-photon microscopy techniques have been applied for deep brain imaging with higher resolution and power of data analysis related to huge valuable information that it could be obtained from high sensitive signaling recorded. For example, in the case of deep-brain three-photon microscopy excited at 1600 nm with silicone oil immersion [16] different gaining media were evaluated, such as D_2O as immersion medium *vs* silicone oil.

These media modification, from aqueous to oil, increased the excitation light transmitted with a 17% enhancement of photon signaling at the 1700 nm window. Silicone oil immersion also enabled 3-photon fluorescence imaging of vasculature up to 1460 μm (mechanical depth) into the mouse brain *in vivo*. This example showed the importance of media and photon interactions. Moreover, by 3-photon fluorescence imaging, demonstration and visualization of astrocytes were reported in the deep mouse brain *in vivo* [17] with Sulforhodamine 101 dye as a fluorescent labeller. Then, fluorescence imaging was performed in astrocytes 910 μm below the surface of the mouse brain *in vivo*, and 30% deeper than using 2-photon fluorescence microscopy. Moreover, through a quantitative comparison of the difference of signals between SR101labeled blood vessels and astrocytes, the challenge of visualizing astrocytes below the white matter was further elucidated.

Also the exploitation of the high sensitive fluorescence lifetime imaging nanoscopy for measuring Förster resonance energy transfer in cellular nanodomains [18] (Fig. **1**). This methodology was adopted in image color mapping and determination of lifetime values for each pixel from the image, multiplied by the corresponding intensity image to record the intensity-weighted lifetime image. Therefore, the resolution of nanodomains of targeted and fluorescent-labelled proteins was determined.

4. MINIATURIZED INSTRUMENTATION FOR *IN VIVO* IMPLANTABLE AND PORTABLE DEVICES

As discussed in the previous sections regarding miniaturized microscopes and optrodes, the valuable data recording *in vivo* has been demonstrated to be really high by portable wireless devices. However, these major technological developments applied to small animals could be extended to humans for advanced health monitoring and precision medicine.

Many developments derived from different technological setups have taken place in order to record different signals at the same time. It could be mentioned the brain stimulation by light application, neural activity recording, molecular and biodetection; and *in vivo* accurate drug delivery depending on needs. Programmable wireless light-emitting diode stimulator for chronic stimulation of optogenetic molecules in freely-moving mice [19] was also reported.

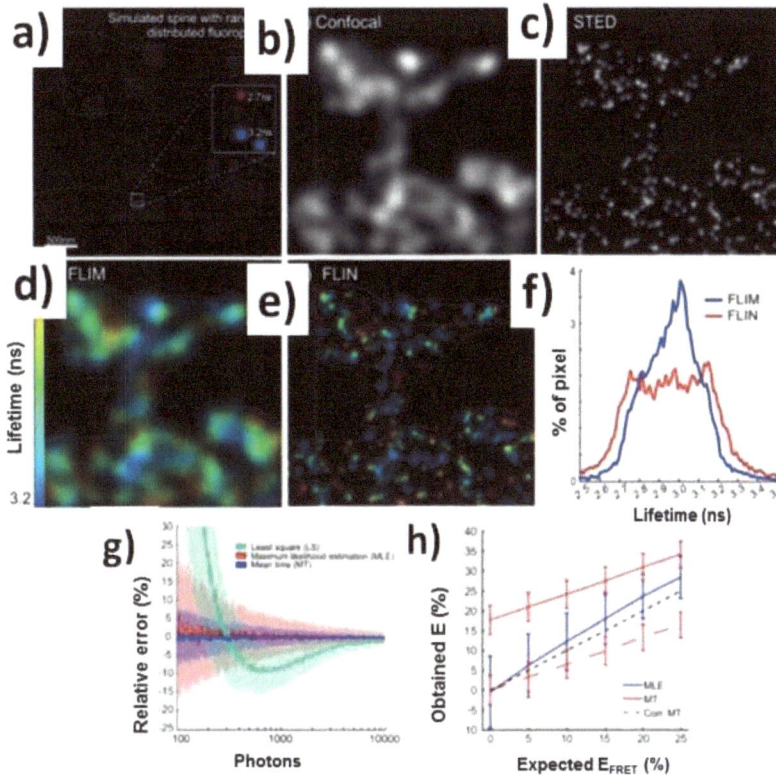

Fig. (1). Simulations of fluorescence lifetime imaging and analysis with diffraction-limited resolution (250 nm; FLIM) or subdiffraction-limited resolution (50 nm; FLIN). [79] Simulated image of randomly positioned fluorescent molecules inside a dendritic spine shape (2.8×2.0 μm) with a lifetime of 3.2ns (donor alone) and 2.7 ns (corresponding to 15% FRET efficiency). (b and c) Simulated confocal (b) and STED (c) intensity image of molecule distribution shown in (a) (FWHM of the simulated PSFs: 250 nm for confocal and 50 nm for STED). (d and e) Simulated FLIM (d) and FLIN (e) intensity-weighted lifetime image obtained by the multiplication of the color-coded lifetime image and the simulated intensity images shown in (b) and (c), respectively. (f) Lifetime distribution for the images shown in (d and e). (g) Relative mean error (±standard deviation, light color) for the fitting algorithm least square (LS), maximum likelihood (MLE) and meantime of photon arrival (MT). (h) Relationship between simulated and ground truth values of FRET efficiency, in the presence of imposed levels of EFRET, using the MT (red), corrected MT (dash red) or MLE (blue) analysis (standard deviation indicated by the error bars). Simulated EFRET is indicated by the dashed black line (correlation of 1.0) [18].

Hence, from miniaturized, multicode, multiband and programmable light-emitting diode (LED) stimulator for wireless control of optogenetic experiments, social and behavioural testing of free rodents was conducted with IR diode photo pulses at different frequencies. In this way, the moving direction of a Thy1-ChR2-YFP transgenic mouse was remotely controlled by transcranially illuminating the corresponding hemisphere of the primary motor-cortex involved.

In addition, splayed optical microfibers [20] were developed to collect individual neural activity. This device consists of an optical fiber array formed by reduced optical fiber sizes of 8 μm, each one for fluorescent signal recording from a small number of non-overlapping neurons near the fiber apertures. Consequently, when the number of fibers increased, the bundle delivered more uniform excitation power to the region, moving to a regime where fibers collected fluorescence from more neurons and greater overlapping was found between neighboring fibers. Under these conditions, it became feasible to apply source separation to gather individual neural information.

A further microdevice for stable neural activity recording was elastocapillary self-assembled neurotassels [21]. This reduced-size device was formed by an array of flexible micro-electrode filament tassel shaped with elastocapillary interactions. These interactions were based on a biocompatible and dissolvable polymer for better neuronal tissue interactions from the diminished surface. Therefore, stable electrical neuronal activities were recorded.

The development of implantable micro-optical devices permitted neural cell analysis [22] and targeted drug delivery applications [23]. Thus, new approaches in Precision Medicine and the development of new personalized treatments could be developed.

This capability to control decreased sizes of instrumentation for signal recording was transferred to *in vivo* neurosurgery in humans, as in the intraoperative detection of blood vessels with an imaging needle [24] (Fig. **2**). This development was motivated based on a particular risk related to intercranial hemorrhages that should be avoided. Thus, optical tomography needle probe in *in vivo* human brain led to the discrimination between blood vessels and tissue. And just to finish it should be highlighted the ethical implications and discussions accompanied with these high impact data recording applications from real implants in humans that they are currently in progress [25].

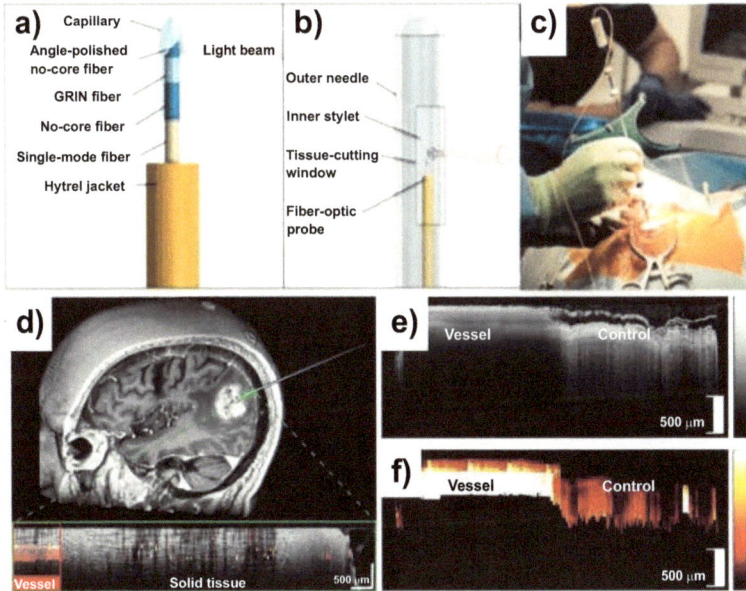

Fig. (2). a) Scheme of the distal end of the fiber optic probe.b) Scheme of the distal end of the imaging needle, showing the outer needle, inner stylet and fiber optic probe. [95] Photo showing the imaging needle inserted into a human brain during surgery (Photo credit: the Audio Visual Production Unit, Sir Charles Gairdner Hospital). d) 3D volume rendered MRI scan showing needle trajectory in a human male brain. e) OCT Scan consisting of A-scans acquired as the needle is manually rolled across the tissue. Tissue surface corresponded to the top of the OCT image, with depth increasing as we move down the image. f) Speckle decorrelation images of vessels and controls from calculations based on OCT scanning [24].

5. NEURO-SIGNALING TRACKING

On the basis of the different spectroscopical techniques, instrumentations and methodologies discussed, many neuro-signaling sources could be tracked. So, it could be tracked variations of biological events that affect to health and behaviour of small animals and humans. Therefore, neuro-hormones, neuro-peptides, neuro-transmitters, biomolecules and inorganic ions could be tracked.

Within all these traceable analytes, we should note the cerebral metabolism in a mouse model of Alzheimer's disease characterized by two-photon fluorescence lifetime microscopy of intrinsic NADH [26]. This fluorescent molecule in the energy metabolism of cells has, generally, played a vital role also in neurons and in the development of many neurodegenerative disorders and cerebral pathologies. Thus, *via* fluorescent signaling, different endogenous fluorescence emissions of reduced nicotinamide adenine dinucleotide (NADH) were recorded *in vivo* correlated with neuro-pathologies. Moreover, the use of molecular sensors for calcium control of neurotransmitter release [27] connected to inter-neuronal signaling has also provided different neuroimaging patterns according to the mental status of rodents, *i.e.,* from calm to stressful situations. For humans, on the other hand, similar studies were performed by non-invasive resonance magnetic imaging [28] (MRI), carried out by the Massachusetts Institute of Technology using a manganese-based MRI contrast agent [29].

The importance of calcium on neuro-modifications was shown by its implication on neuro-inflammatory processes as well. For instance, the neuronal S100B protein showed a calcium-tuning suppression of amyloid-beta-aggregation [30] (Fig. **3**) in the Alzheimer's disease development as well as in inflammatory brain processes. The Amyloid-β (Aβ) aggregation and neuro-inflammation are consistent features in Alzheimer's disease (AD) and strong candidates for the initiation of neurodegeneration. S100B is one of the most abundant pro-inflammatory proteins that are chronically up-regulated in AD and found to be associated with senile plaques. This recognized biomarker for brain distress may, thus, play a central role in amyloid aggregation, which remains to be determined. In this context, a novel role for the neuronal S100B protein as a suppressor of Aβ 42 aggregation and toxicity was reported.

This effect was observed from the determination of the structural details of the interaction between monomeric Aβ 42 and S100B, which is favored by calcium-binding to S100B, possibly involving conformational switching of disordered Aβ into an α-helical conformer, which locked aggregation. This physical interaction was coupled with a functional role in the inhibition of Aβ 42 aggregation and toxicity, and this phenomenon was modified by calcium binding to S100B.

As previously discussed, with these examples, the neuro signal tracking showed a high impact from the analytical viewpoint due to the intrinsic channel of signal discrimination, summed to the conclusions obtained from the recorded signals. Other examples could also be discussed in relation to another biomolecular tracking; however, they fall outside the scope of this section. Here, we intend to show the importance of these techniques and methodologies within neuroscience and neurophotonics.

From the area of neuroscience, many developments are currently in progress in numerous technological fields. For example it could be focused on biomimetic designs, such as the fabrication of photonic on-chip synapses [31], potentially extended to other micro- and nanodevice applications (Fig. **4**).

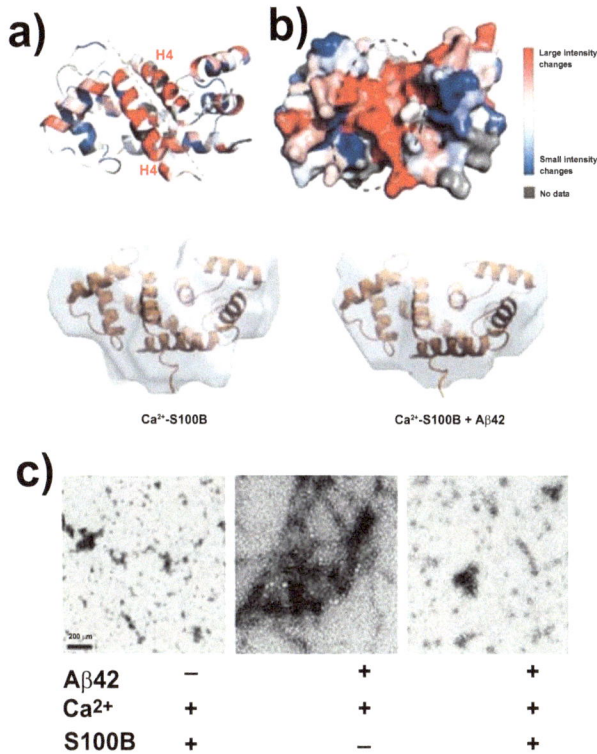

Fig. (3). a) Structure of Ca^{2+}-S100B [Protein Data Bank (PDB) code: 2H61], color-coded by the degree of difference in peak intensity in the absence or presence of Aβ42. Unassigned residues are colored gray, while residues that correspond to peaks that undergo large intensity changes are colored red, and residues that correspond to peaks that change little or not at all are colored blue, with a gradient for values in between. Left: Ribbon representation. Dashed line indicates the interfacial cleft. Right: Surface representation at the same orientation. Dashed circle highlights the putative Aβ42 binding region. **b)** SAXS-based structural model of S100B in the absence (left) and in the presence (right) of Aβ42, both in the presence of calcium. The surface represents the best SAXS models based on the fit between the experimental data and the back-calculated SAXS data and have been overlapped with the experimental NMR structure (PDB code: 2K7O). **c)** TEM images with a nanogold-conjugated secondary antibody against S100B (15 nm) and Aβ42 (10 nm), showing binding of S100B to fibrils and oligomers [30].

This photonic approach looked for new neuromorphic computing systems for signal transduction and storage, such as a biomimetic device of neuronal synapsis in the brain based on the design of a hardware device *via* a photonic integrated-circuit approach. This device was created on modified and integrated silicon nitride waveguides with a phase change material in order to emulate the neuro synapsis that allowed varying the optical pulses sent down through the waveguides, resulting in ultrafast operation speed, virtually unlimited bandwidth and no electrical interconnect-power loss.

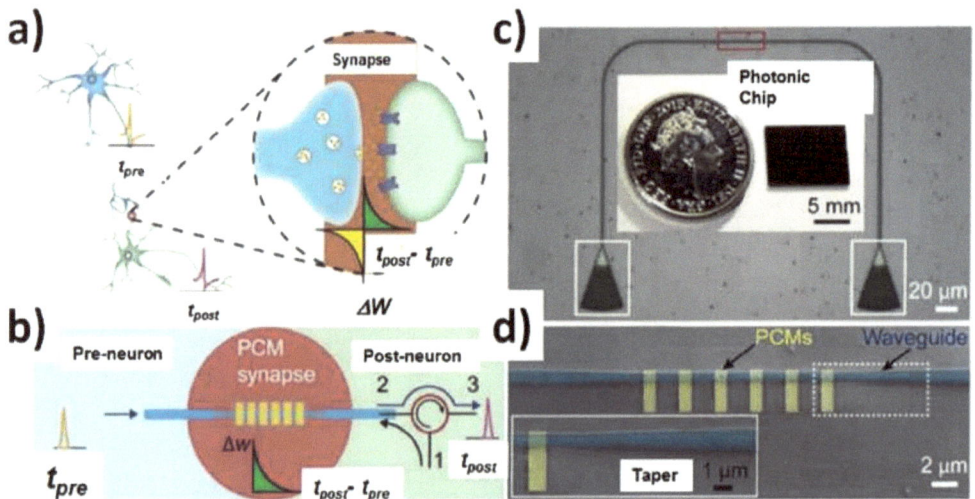

Fig. (4). On-chip photonic synapse. **a)** Structure of neuron and synapse. Inset: Illustration of the synapse junction. **b)** Scheme of the integrated photonic synapse resembling the function of the neural synapse. The synapse is based on a tapered waveguide (dark blue) with discrete phase change material (PCM) islands on top, optically connecting the presynaptic (pre-neuron) and the postsynaptic (post-neuron) signals. The red open circle is a circulator with port 2 and port 3 connecting the synapse and the post-neuron; weighting pulses are applied through port 1 to the synapse. **c)** Optical microscope image of a device with the active region (red box) as the photonic synapse. The optical input to and output from the device are *via* apodized diffractive couplers (white boxes). Inset: A typical photonic chip containing 70 photonic synapses has a dimension smaller than a 5-pence coin. **d)** Scanning electron microscope image of the active region of the photonic synapse corresponding to the red box in (c) with six GST units (1 mm×3 mm, yellow, false-colored) on top of the waveguide (blue, false-colored). Inset: The zoomed-in tapered structure of the waveguide highlighted by the white dashed box [31].

CONCLUDING REMARKS

From neurophotonics, high valuable results with impact on the knowledge generation about animal behaviour, neurophysiology and neurodegenerative health problems such as Alzheimer could be yielded. At this point, it should be highlighted that the level of knowledge could be generated from small animals to humans. In this manner, data collection from moving animals in vivo has increased substantially due to the implementation of implantable and portable devices. Therefore, based on these devices could be developed by many neurological studies. For example, contemplating from interaction with the environment with biological implications to invasive drug effects accompanied with tracking of neuro-active molecules or generating neuroimaging.

REFERENCES

[1]   B. Blanco, M. Molnar, and C. Caballero-Gaudes, "Effect of prewhitening in resting-state functional near-infrared spectroscopy data", *Neurophoton,* vol. 5, no. 040401, pp. 1-14, 2018.

[2]   S. Bloch, F. Lesage, A. Gandjbakhche, and K. Liang, "Whole-body fluorescence lifetime imaging of a tumortargeted near-infrared molecular probe in mice", *Journal of Biomedical Optics,* vol. 10, no. 054003, pp. 1-7, 2005.

[3]   O. Gliko, G. D. Reddy, W. E. Brownell, and P. Saggau, "Standing wave total internal reflection fluorescence microscopy to measure the size of nanostructures in living cells", *Journal of Biomedical Optics,* vol. 11, no. 064013, pp. 1-5, 2006.

[4]   S. Skinner, *Reprinted from Australian Familly Physician,* vol. 42, no. 11, pp. 794-797, 2013.

[5]   J. Yao, and L. V. Wang, "Photoacoustic brain imaging: from microscopic to macroscopic scales", *Neurophotonics,* vol. 1, no. 011003, p. 1.13, 2014.

[6]   D. A. Boas, and A. K. Dunn, "Laser speckle contrast imaging in biomedical optics", *Journal of Biomedical Optics,* vol. 15, no. 01110, pp. 1-12, 2010.

[7]   W. Ren, H. Skulason, F. Schlegel, M. Rudin, J. Klohs, and R. Ni, "Automated registration of magnetic resonance imaging and optoacoustic tomography data for experimental studies", *Neurophoton,* vol. 6, no. 025001, pp. 1-10, 2019.

[8]   K. Sugino, C.M. Hempel, M.N. Miller, A.M. Hattox, P. Shapiro, C. Wu, Z.J. Huang, and S.B. Nelson, "Molecular taxonomy of major neuronal classes in the adult mouse forebrain", *Nat. Neurosci.,* vol. 9, no. 1, pp. 99-107, 2006.
[http://dx.doi.org/10.1038/nn1618] [PMID: 16369481]

[9]   N. Vogt, *Neuron,* vol. 98, pp. 905-917, 2018.
[http://dx.doi.org/10.1016/j.neuron.2018.05.028] [PMID: 29879392]

[10]   C.M. Hempel, K. Sugino, and S.B. Nelson, "A manual method for the purification of fluorescently labeled neurons from the mammalian brain", *Nat. Protoc.,* vol. 2, no. 11, pp. 2924-2929, 2007.
[http://dx.doi.org/10.1038/nprot.2007.416] [PMID: 18007629]

[11]   A.C. Cuello, J.V. Priestley, and M.V. Sofroniew, "Immunocytochemistry and neurobiology", *Q. J. Exp. Physiol.,* vol. 68, no. 4, pp. 545-578, 1983.
[http://dx.doi.org/10.1113/expphysiol.1983.sp002748] [PMID: 6139841]

[12]   Z. Pode, R. Peri-Naor, J.M. Georgeson, T. Ilani, V. Kiss, T. Unger, B. Markus, H.M. Barr, L. Motiei, and D. Margulies, "Protein recognition by a pattern-generating fluorescent molecular probe", *Nat. Nanotechnol.,* vol. 12, no. 12, pp. 1161-1168, 2017.
[http://dx.doi.org/10.1038/nnano.2017.175] [PMID: 29035400]

[13]   L. Bezin, D. Marcel, L.I. Debure, N. Ginovart, and C. Rousset, J. Frangois Pujol, and D. Weissmann, "Postnatal development of the tyrosine hydroxylase-containing cell population within the rat locus coeruleus: topological organization and phenotypic plasticity", *J. Neurosci.,* vol. 14, no. 12, pp. 7488-7501, 1994.
[http://dx.doi.org/10.1523/JNEUROSCI.14-12-07486.1994]

[14]   C. O'Connor, "Fluorescence in situ hybridization (FISH)", *Nature Education,* vol. 1, no. 1, pp. 171-173, 2008.

[15]   L. Amirav, S. Berlin, S. Olszakier, S.K. Pahari, and I. Kahn, "Multi-modal nano particle labeling of neurons", *Front. Neurosci.,* vol. 13, no. 12, p. 12, 2019.
[http://dx.doi.org/10.3389/fnins.2019.00012] [PMID: 30778281]

[16]   S. Tong, H. Liu, H. Cheng, C. He, Y. Du, Z. Zhuang, P. Qiu, and K. Wang, "Deep-brain three-photon microscopy excited at 1600 nm with silicone oil immersion", *J. Biophotonics,* vol. 12, no. 6, p. e201800423, 2019.
[http://dx.doi.org/10.1002/jbio.201800423] [PMID: 30801979]

[17]   H. Liu, J. Wang, Z. Zhuang, J. He, W. Wen, P. Qiu, and K. Wang, "Visualizing astrocytes in the deep mouse brain *in vivo.*", *J. Biophotonics,* vol. 12, no. 7, p. e201800420, 2019.

[http://dx.doi.org/10.1002/jbio.201800420] [PMID: 30938095]

[18]   C. Tardif, G. Nadeau, S. Labrecque, D. Côté, F. Lavoie-Cardina, and P. De Koninck, "Fluorescence lifetime imaging nanoscopy for measuring Förster resonance energy transfer in cellular nanodomains", *Neurophoton,* vol. 6, no. 015002, pp. 1-16, 2019.

[19]   M. Hashimoto, A. Hata, T. Miyata, and H. Hirase, "Programmable wireless light-emitting diode stimulator for chronic stimulation of optogenetic molecules in freely moving mice", *Neurophotonics,* vol. 1, no. 011002, pp. 1-10, 2019.

[20]   L. N. Perkins, A. Devor, T. J. Gardner, and D. A. Boas, "Extracting individual neural activity recorded through splayed optical microfibers", *Neurophoton,* vol. 5, no. 5, pp. 1-10, 2018.

[21]   S. Guan, J. Wang, X. Gu, Y. Zhao, R. Hou, H. Fan, L. Zou, L. Gao, M. Du, C. Li, and Y. Fang, "Elastocapillary self-assembled neurotassels for stable neural activity recording", *Sci. Adv,* vol. 5, no. eaav2842, pp. 1-11, 2019.

[22]   H. Takehara, A. Nagaoka, J. Noguchi, T. Akagi, H. Kasai, and T. Ichiki, "Lab-on-a-brain: implantable micro-optical fluidic devices for neural cell analysis *in vivo*", *Sci. Rep.,* vol. 4, no. 6721, p. 6721, 2014. [PMID: 25335545]

[23]   C.M. Proctor, A. Slézia, A. Kaszas, A. Ghestem, I. Del Agua, A.M. Pappa, C. Bernard, A. Williamson, and G.G. Malliaras, "Electrophoretic drug delivery for seizure control", *Sci. Adv.,* vol. 4, no. 8, p. eaau1291, 2018.
[http://dx.doi.org/10.1126/sciadv.aau1291] [PMID: 30167463]

[24]   H. Ramakonar, B. C. Quirk, R. W. Kirk, J. Li, A. Jacques, C. R. P. Lind, and R. A. McLaughlin, "Intraoperative detection of blood vessels with an imaging needle during neurosurgery in humans", *Sci. Adv,* vol. 4, no. eaav4992, pp. 1-10, 2018.

[25]   E. Underwood, "Researchers grapple with the ethics of testing brain implants, Brain & Behavior", *Sci. Commun.,* vol. 1-2, 2017.
[http://dx.doi.org/10.1126/science.aar3698]

[26]   C. A. Gómez, B. Fu, S. Sakadžic, and M. A. Yaseen, "Cerebral metabolism in a mouse model of Alzheimer's disease characterized by two-photon fluorescence lifetime microscopy of intrinsic NADH", *Neurophoton,* vol. 5, no. 045008, pp. 1-6, 2018.

[27]   T.C. Südhof, "Calcium control of neurotransmitter release", *Cold Spring Harb. Perspect. Biol.,* vol. 4, no. 1, p. a011353, 2012.
[http://dx.doi.org/10.1101/cshperspect.a011353] [PMID: 22068972]

[28]   J. Duyn, and A.P. Koretsky, "Magnetic resonance imaging of neural circuits", *Nat. Clin. Pract. Cardiovasc. Med.,* vol. 5, suppl. Suppl. 2, pp. S71-S78, 2008.
[http://dx.doi.org/10.1038/ncpcardio1248] [PMID: 18641610]

[29]   A. Barandov, B.B. Bartelle, C.G. Williamson, E.S. Loucks, S.J. Lippard, and A. Jasanoff, "Sensing intracellular calcium ions using a manganese-based MRI contrast agent", *Nat. Commun.,* vol. 10, no. 1, p. 897, 2019.
[http://dx.doi.org/10.1038/s41467-019-08558-7] [PMID: 30796208]

[30]   J. S. Cristóvão, V. K. Morris, I. Cardoso, S. S. Leal, J. Martínez, H. M. Botelho, C. Göbl, R. David, K. Kierdorf, M. Alemi, T. Madl, G. Fritz, B. Reif, and C. M. Gomes, "The neuronal S100B protein is a calcium-tuned suppressor of amyloid-beta-aggregation", *Sci. Adv,* vol. 4, no. eaaq1702, pp. 1-13, 2018.

[31]   Z. Cheng, C. Ríos, W.H.P. Pernice, C.D. Wright, and H. Bhaskaran, "On-chip photonic synapse", *Sci. Adv.,* vol. 3, no. 9, p. e1700160, 2017.
[http://dx.doi.org/10.1126/sciadv.1700160] [PMID: 28959725]

CHAPTER 14

Precision Nanomedicine Based on Genomics and Drug Delivery Systems

Abstract: Precision nanomedicine based on advanced diagnosis by personalized analysis with, for example, the incorporation of genomics and specific biomarker tracking have allowed faster diagnosis and application of treatments. With controlled-size cargo nanoparticles, potential applications were also devised for targeted drug delivery, in addition to new enzymatic approaches addressing targeted delivery for targeted DNA repairs. Another novel gene therapy is also discussed. Moreover, we show, for personalized drug assay tests, how design-led to bioassays within microfluidic four-organ-chip devices in order to evaluate compatibilities and effects according to the nature and response of the organism.

Keywords: CRISPR-Cas9, Drug delivery system, Genomics, Gene therapy, Implantable microdevice, Lab-on particle, Precision nanomedicine, Personalized medicine.

1. INTRODUCTION

For precision medicine, advanced diagnosis and personalized analysis need to be discussed in order to examine/explore individual biological variations in specific health problems or biological systems. Only then it will be possible to apply the effective treatment. In order to arrive to this level of health care for targeted applications, accurate clinical analysis should be conducted from biological markers and genomics, where major challenges should be responded to. From the viewpoint of clinical analysis, the use of small quantities of real samples with faster and lower limits needs to be still addressed to advance the accurate point-of-care diagnosis.

Therefore, through the most effective treatment, prevention should be aimed at decreasing treatment time and avoiding undesirable secondary effects. There are thus numerous developments from fundamental science with potential transference for incorporation within instruments. These instrumental set - ups could be applied in life sciences as well as in other fields where specialrequirements are needed. At this point, it should be mentioned that these types of developments were done by the use of multidisciplinary knowledge accompanied with a long vision of the future.

These technologies are in progress, demonstrating the importance of different nanoarchitecture designs by its incorporation to improve existing methodologies (Fig. **1**). Therefore, we should consider the control of the nanoscale for nanotechnological developments such as lab-on particles and lab-on chips, in conjunction with genomics and a faster-miniaturized gene detection, as well as with metabolomics and bimolecular tracking that could allow the application of the most effective treatment.

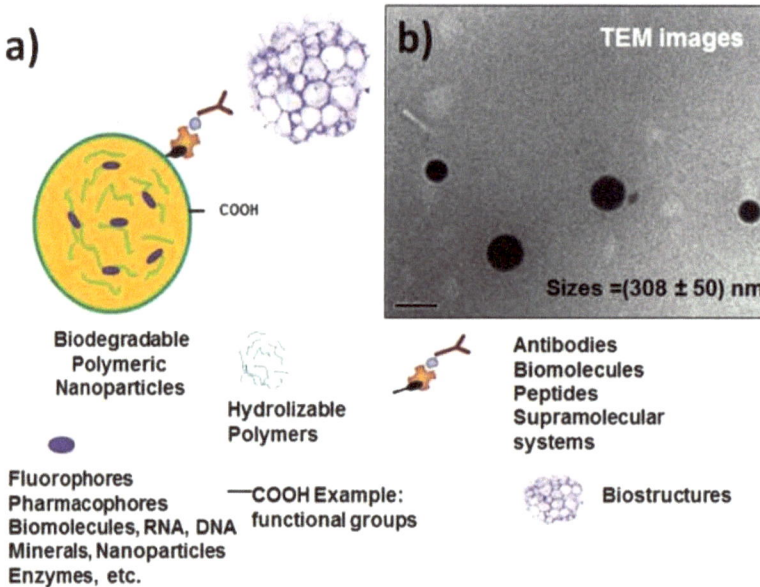

Fig. (1). a) Schematic representation of cargo-loaded nanoparticles for tracking and drug delivery applications. **b)** TEM images of organic biodegradable nanoparticles.

These treatments should be properly controlled and tracked, for example, withcontrolled drug delivery and tracking of the desired effect. In this field, advanced switchable cargo nanoparticle developments and multifunctional implantable devices have been reported, and by advanced gene therapies in progress based on biocompatible and degradable nanoparticles (Fig. **1**).

At the moment the state of the art of these types of Nanoarchitectures arrived to be tested from small animals as rodents, monkeys and even to human's trials.

Hence, this section intends to review the main and most recent studies with perspectives in the near future.

2. NEW ADVANCED DIAGNOSIS BASED ON LAB-ON PARTICLES

In this respect, the concept of lab-on particles based on the appropriate development of a functional particle used as a platform for specific molecular detection, drug delivery and another particular functionalities required for faster diagnosis is highly required for low **LODs** at the single-molecule level of detection and targeted delivery. The interactions of these multifunctional particles could be tracked and controlled by different optical detection systems. The concept can be easily understood; however, their development posed challenges that should be overcome. For biomolecular detection, specific recognition, detection and quantification *in vivo* or from cleaned-up samples were shown to be the greatest challenge; thus a targeted treatment was adopted. Many spectroscopical signals could be tracked; yet, for a given specific analyte, possibilities are often reduced depending on their intrinsic properties or complex matrixes into where they are incorporated. For these reasons, molecular, biomolecular and biostructure labelling could be used as a direct or an indirect pathway of detection.

For example, plasmonic fluorescence enhancement by metal-nanostructures could shape the future of bio-nanotechnology and bioassays [1]. These developments based on the **MEF** effect previously discussed have allowed, for instance, increased bioassay sensitivity of bioactive molecules using induced metal-enhanced bioluminescence [2] by tuning the plasmonic nanoarchitectures for specific fluorescent analyte incorporated in bacteria membranes. In this research bioluminescence signal enhancement was done *via* proximity based on the deposition of a tuned plasmonic silver nanoparticle for a targeted fluorescent bioactive compound detection. This approach employed a whole-cell bioreporter harboring a plasmid-borne fusion of a specific promoter incorporated with a bioluminescence reporter gene. To develop this methodology, first, it was optimized the silver deposition process of optimal nanoparticle sizes for the targeted application.

Silver deposition of 350 nm particles enabled the doubling of the bioluminescent signal amplitude by the bacterial bio-reporter when compared to an untouched non-silver-deposited microtiter plate surface. Thus, a proof of concept demonstrated to have potential applications that could be extended to other targeted molecules incorporated in biostructures based on a nanoplatform as a nanosensor, only detected in the presence of the fluorescent reporter incorporated in the bio-membrane.

During the last two decades, facilitating the provision of red blood cell units to allo-immunized patients has been seen as a major development in genotyping assays. In order to make genotyping faster, simpler and less costly, a nanotechnology approach was designed from silver metal/silica fluorescent nanoparticles. This nanoarchitecture linked to the development of enhanced fluorescence detection based on plasmonic nanoplatforms for **MEF** genotyping [3] was done by the appropriate design of silver nanoparticles. The nanoparticles were optimized by the addition of silica spacer shells for **MEF** of an energy acceptor/emitter placed at the right distance. Then, this **MEF** nanoplatform was modified with the targeted DNA strand non-covalent grafted with a low fluorescent polymer that became optically active upon hybridization with the targeted complementary DNA strand. Based on this free PCR DNA nanoplatform, direct molecular detection of SRY gene was achieved from unamplified genomic DNA by **MEF** and **FRET** and validated for free PCR analysis of SRY gene in real blood samples [4, 5].

Thus, it was shown how functional or multifunctional nanoplatforms such as lab-on particle could be designed for biomolecular detection and required treatments. Such requirements include molecular or biostructure recognition, signal transductions, enhanced signaling based on nano-approaches for single molecules or low number of analytes per nanoplatform detected, with the possibility of including in-flow methodologies, microchips, and microdevices. In addition, it should note the importance of single nanoplatform tracking *in vivo* from where the specific region of detection or action of a given functionality could be known/determined.

3. LAB-ON CHIPS

Currently, a large number of research fields have applied the miniaturization on chips available. Concerning lab-on chips for bioassay applications, confined compartments from the accurate patterning of different polymeric materials were used. As for example, such as glass, modified siloxane and metamaterials with different designs, channels and waveguides, allowed the incorporation of multiple steps for sample manipulation, clean-up and coupled signal transduction.

These patterns of materials could be developed through different techniques by applying high-energy power of lasers, electronic beams. Thus, the different topographies in the Nanoscale could be modified by multilayer deposition of different materials in order to develop their specific functionalities. Cases of this include multi-organ-on-chips for long-term biomedical investigations [6]. These systems were designed to minimize costs, manipulate smaller real samples or monitor in real-time different physical and chemical variables that could even be used to mimic the *in vivo* environments and be applied on drug delivery, toxicity and molecular tracking tests (Fig. **2**). In order to develop these microfluidic devices, we should refer to the use of polycarbonate cover-plates, PDMS-glass chip with varying dimensions, coupled to real sample inlets, and excretory flow circuits.

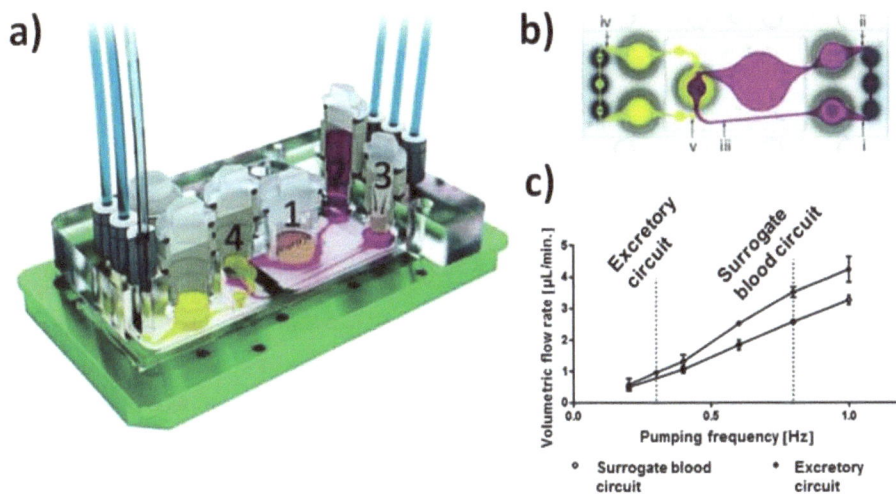

Fig. (2). The microfluidic four-organ-chip device at a glance. **a)** 3D view of the device, comprising two polycarbonate cover-plates, the PDMS-glass chip (footprint: 76 mm × 25 mm; height: 3 mm) accommodating a surrogate blood flow circuit (pink) and an excretory flow circuit (yellow). Numbers represent the four tissue culture compartments for the intestine (1), liver (2), skin (3) and kidneys (4). A central cross-section of each tissue culture compartment aligned along the interconnecting microchannel is depicted.
b) Evaluation of fluid dynamics in the 4OC using μPIV (micro-scale particle image velocimetry, an optical method of flow visualization used to obtain instantaneous velocity measurements and related properties in fluids in microscale). Top view of the four-organ-chip layout, illustrating the positions of three measuring spots (i, ii, and iii) in the surrogate blood circuit and two spots (iv, v) in the excretory circuit. **c)** Average volumetric flow rate plotted against the pumping frequency of the surrogate blood flow circuit and the excretory circuit. Co-culture experiments were performed at 0.8 Hz and 0.3 Hz, respectively, as indicated by the vertical lines. Error bars are the standard error of the mean [6].

In addition these devices designed as organ on-chips could be mimetized as in interconnected tissue culture compartments like intestine, liver, skin and kidneys. Thus, targeted signaling by coupling appropriate detection systems could be recorded, such as multimodal imaging and the different detection strategies previously discussed.

Hence, the lab-on particles could be applied in high-potential real applications for molecular profiling in precision medicine oncology [7] and innovative analysis beyond DNA sequencing, such as epigenetic analysis, RNA sequencing and proteomic assessment. In this respect, substantial advances can be made by combining multidisciplinary fields, such as genomic and transcriptomic profiling that expanded precision cancer medicine known as WINTHER trial, recently developed by France, Spain, Israel, Canada and the United States [8]. The WINTHER trial (NCT01856296) used patients to therapy on the basis of fresh biopsy-derived DNA sequencing (arm A; 236 gene panel) or RNA expression (arm B; comparing tumor to normal). The clinical management committee of researchers from five countries recommended therapies, prioritizing genomic matches, and physicians specified the therapy administered. Human trials were experimentally designed accurately; yet, from the methodology used, we should note the gene profiling performed *via* oligo-array technology with a compressive full human gene expression developed by well-known companies available on the market (Agilent inkjet printing 8 × 60k oligo-arrays).

With oligo-arrays, further research is required for surface modification with targeted single-stranded DNA and RNA in order to develop microarrays [9]. Additionally, in order to improve these methodologies, these research fields could be expanded and incorporated into the design of lab-on particles and lab-on chips.

Thus, the different developed nanosensor could be incorporated as implantable as well as portable devices. By this manner specific analytes, and biostructures obtained from cleaned up real samples and non-processed matrixes could be analyzed.

4. GENOMICS AND MINIATURIZED ANALYSIS

As it is well known the gene profiling is very important to be in advance in recognition of specific expressions related with behaviours and different states of health. Currently, the polymeric chain reaction (**PCR**) is the most widely used and recognized assay applied to human clinical analysis. However, some challenges need to be faced, which has motivated researchers to develop new methodologies, such as quantitative fluorescence polymerase chain reaction (QF-PCR) and fluorescence *in situ* hybridization (FISH) [10], both largely tested and validated in real samples [11]. Yet, some variables need to be improved, as in the case of lower costs, sample volumes and total time required for the whole analysis. Hence, further approaches are being designed in order to overcome these problems in the area of microdevices and micro-chips such as microfluidics chips designs, due to their reduced size and smaller real sample volumes requirements.As an introduction, within microdevices and miniaturized approaches, the design of multi-chamber microfluidic chips for coupled compartmentalized multi-functionalities is important in the clinical analysis of red-blood gene expression, where multi-step methodologies should be applied. Thus, multiplexed enrichment and genomic profiling of peripheral blood cells revealed subset-specific immune signatures [12]. In order to study that, a low-input microfluidic system was designed for sorting immune cells into subsets and profiling their gene expression. A two-layer microfluidic device is? capable of semi-automated cell isolation, cell disruption and sequence library construction protocols. This system integrates microfluidic liquid handling withmagnetic affinity purification and capability for onboard polymerase chain reaction (PCR). The device was developed by a two-layer soft lithography technique. It consisted of an operating unit formed by three main chambers connected to pneumatic valve controllers to handle mammalian cell samples. The largest chamber was rectangular, used for cell isolation, while the two smaller "rotary reactor" chambers were used for gene library recording. These reactors were fitted with internal microvalves are used to formulate sample and reagent combinations. In addition, reduced-size magnets were added in order to move the magnetic beads from one chamber to others and silicon wafer surfaces for accurate temperature control according to the requirements of the bioanalysis step.

In this way, subset-specific disease signatures were identified by profiling four immune cell subsets in blood from patients with systemic lupus erythematosus (SLE) and matched control subjects by using low RNA inputs. In this development, it should be highlighted that the analysis was performed from low number of cells within a cm scale device.

In addition, it could be mentioned the development of portable infrared isothermal **PCR** platform for multiple sexually transmitted diseases by strand detection [13] within a multichamber microfluidic chip as well, but with the incorporation of IR light-emitting diode devices (**LED**) for accurate temperature control. This microfluidic chip integrated the RNA extraction, micropump and multi-target detection onto the same chip of 13x15x7 cm, allowing a fulfilled isothermal amplification in 70 min. This platform enabled the detection of weak fluorescence emissions from multiplexed pathogen signaling.

In addition, **SMD** approaches based on nanoimaging for dynamic studies at selectively single-molecule level within gene transcriptions [14]. Thus, the potential of bioanalysis, in conjunction with the development of microdevices, shows potential for multiple applications.

5.   TARGETED   DRUG,   CARGO   NANOPARTICLES   AND IMPLANTABLE DEVICES FOR CONTROLLED ADMINISTRATION

Targeted drug delivery for precision medicine applications has many challenges to respond to. Assuming that one of the main factors has already been overcome, in relation to the efficiency and specificity of the drug for a given treatment, the way of administration should also be evaluated. Hence, from small molecules to cargo nanoparticles many barriers should be reduced to arrive at the specific cell. For these reasons different types of nanoarchitectures and biomaterials have been developed and are currently being evaluated on the basis of varying strategies. For instance, in connection with new ways of administration, smart nanodrug administration with nuclear localization sequences in the presence of MMP-2 is worth mentioning to overcome bio-barriers and drug resistance [15]. Based on prolonged circulation lifetime and enhanced accumulation of drug at the tumor site *via* enhanced permeability and retention effect, nanoparticle-based drug formulations for cancer treatments can overcome/remove pharmacokinetic limitations associated with conventional drug formulations. However, due to the complex matrix where cancer cells are placed, the tumor microenvironment has plenty/numerous physiological barriers against cargo nanoparticles, such as elevated interstitial fluid pressure and dense interstitial matrix. Such physiological barriers severely hinder the penetration and diffusion of these types of nanoparticles in tumors. Furthermore, phagocytosis systems and organelle trapping during the path to the targeted cell should also be taken into account. Therefore, all these variables should be evaluated and tested in terms of drug resistance and real effect *in vivo*. Moreover, nanoparticles size and surface modification could affect interactions and effect as well. For example large 100 nm nanoparticles are desired for cargo drug delivery applications, while smaller sizes such as 10 nm are more suitable for diffusion in tumor interstitium [16].

Moreover, from all the possible ways of administration, injectable applications showed enhanced delivery for cancer therapeutics [17], based on the micrometer-sized particle of loaded poly (L-glutamic acid) polymer with chemotherapeutic drugs such as doxorubicin. These nanoparticles showed to be pH sensitive, with a cleavable linker, which could spontaneously form nanometer-sized particles in an aqueous solution suitable to be transported to the perinuclear region. In this way, metastatic breast cancer showed functional cure in 40–50% of treated mice.

Regarding biomaterial used for drug delivery nanoparticles, all these materials should be biocompatible for the detection of biological events and cell tracking and required treatments. Polymeric nanoparticles, core-shell nanoparticles, and nano supramolecular nanoparticles provide many possibilities to develop and optimize their application [18]. Biodegradable nanoparticles made by many monomers can also be considered, such as poly-lactic acid (PLA) [19], poly-glycolic acid (PGA) and co-polymers formed by both monomers (PLGA) [20, 21]; they are the most biocompatible materials [22] for drug delivery applications and others such as poly-lactic malic co-polymers (PLMA) [23] synthesised applied as shells in nanostructures.

Another strategy applied for different treatments that could be mentioned in the application of immunochemistry for targeted biostructures applications in order to modify biological processes as cancer cell developments or cell deaths. As for example immunotherapy such as immune checkpoint blockade, which enhanced the systemic adaptive immune response, may have potential in combating neurodegeneration, however some reports showed that it failed, and raising questions about the effectiveness of this approach [24]. But it is well known many other applications where the immunochemistry showed to be very useful from cancer cell targeting [25] to drug delivery applications [26].

In case of treatments beyond the biostructures generated, new treatment actions should be discussed at a genomic level. For example, to create a new RNA-based therapy to correct aberrant endothelial cell gene expression in humans, efficient gene silencing in the endothelium of nonhuman primates was achieved by delivering small interfering RNA (siRNA) using ionisable low-molecular weight polymeric nanoparticles [27]. Similarly, we could refer to the use of perfluoroalkyl bicyclic cell-penetrating peptides for delivery of antisense oligonucleotides [28] in the nucleus (Fig. **3**).

New approaches of biomolecule protection should also be reported for improved targeted delivery as evidence of RNAi in humans from systemically administered siRNA *via* nanoparticle Nanoplatform. This Nanoarchitecture was developed with the incorporation of supramolecular systems such as cyclodextrins (cyclic oligosaccharides of glucose) [29]. By this manner, the transport of nucleoside triphosphates into cells by artificial molecular transporters were targeted based on strong non-covalent interactions between ATP and modified cyclodextrins on Nanoparticles [30].

Then, from microfluidic technology, multiple designs of microfluidic approaches were developed for controlled-free drug delivery, as well as drug encapsulated within cargo nanoparticles; their encapsulation in droplets of different size led to in-flow methodologies. Moreover, the design of microneedles coupled to microfluidics also resulted in injections and controlled delivery of low volumes of pharmacophores, drugs and cargo nanoparticles [31]. A case in point is the electrophoretic drug delivery for seizure control [32], consisting of an implantable microfluidic channel connected to respective pumps and coupled to an electrochemical sensor. This device was implanted on a rodent in order to record electrochemical signaling from stimulated voltage gated K channel by local injection of 4-aminopyridine (4AP) into the hippocampus of anesthetized mice for epilepsy induction to evaluate potential drug delivery applications. Consequently, the probe could detect pathological activity and then intervene to stop seizures by delivering inhibitory neurotransmitters directly to the seizure source (Fig. **4**).

Similarly, this functionality could be extended to lab-on-a-brain implantable micro-optical fluidic devices for neural cell analysis *in vivo* [33] potentially implemented in personalized and precision medicine.

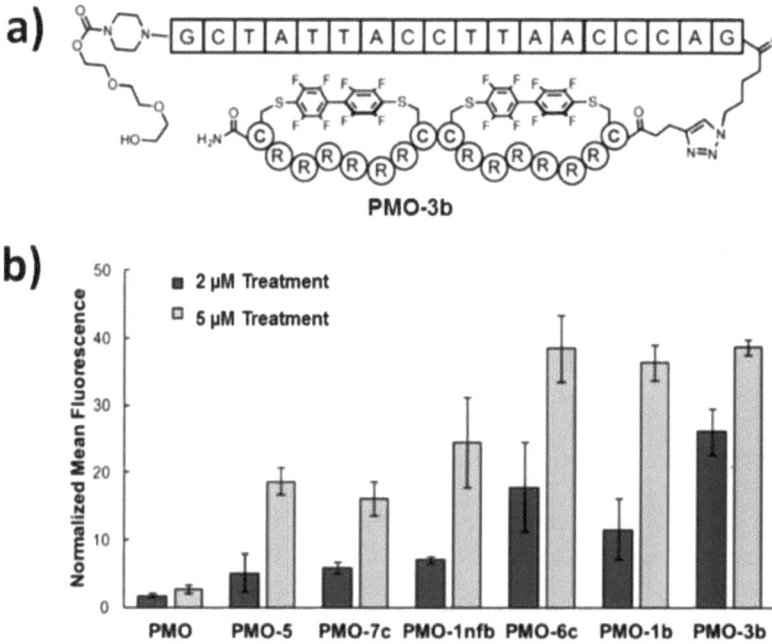

Fig. (3). a) Bicyclic peptides conjugated to phosphorodiamidate morpholino oligonucleotides (PMOs) show increased exon-skipping activity. a) Depiction of bicyclic peptide conjugate PMO-3b. **b)** Conjugates between PMO and perfluoro-aryl cyclic or bicyclic peptides (3b, 5, 7c, nfb, 6c, b correspond to different conjugated peptides) lead to more cellular fluorescence than conjugates to a linear R12 (5), an established cyclic peptide cR10 (7c) or anon-fluorinated bicyclic peptide (1nfb). The PMO corrects eGFP splicing in a modified HeLa cell line. Cells were incubated with 2 [25]. or 5 mm of each PMO-peptide conjugate for 22 h and the mean fluorescence intensity was analyzed by flow cytometry. Error bars are standard deviation (n=3 independent replicates) [28].

To encourage drug and nanotechnology developments, it should be noted the importance of multidisciplinary discussions from basic nanomedicine to applied research aimed at human trials in order to evaluate real developments of products. In these types of Research studies, researchers and governments should discuss in advance long-term objectives depending on needs [34].

6. GENE THERAPIES AND NEW TARGETED DELIVERY SYSTEMS

In the last years precision medicine has focused on genomic treatments with the arrival of the clustered regularly interspaced short palindromic repeat methodology for gene editing, known as CRISPR. Basically CRISPR consisted of the enzymatic DNA cutting as biological scissors incorporating a targeted single DNA strand assayed at different *in vitro* and *in vivo* levels from cells and small animals to humans [35]. In order to discuss this theme, we should refer to the most representative examples and advances in the field. For example, the value of this methodology was shown in dogs by CRISPR, fixing specific muscular dystrophy [36]. The genome-editing tool introduced a mutation in a dog gene that, in effect, overrode a mutation responsible for a disease that mimics Duchenne muscular dystrophy (DMD). As a result, muscle cells in the dogs began to produce the dystrophin protein in many tissues. Moreover, this targeted gene editing methodology proved to pave the way for the development of monkey models that mimic human diseases [37]. This was the first evidence that CRISPR could work in primates, representing a major advance over previous developments in genetically-modified monkey tissues. Then, humans have been injected with gene-editing tools to cure a rare metabolic disorder called Hunter syndrome [38]. The Hunter syndrome results from a mutation in a gene that express an enzyme that cells need it to break down certain sugars. When the enzyme is defective or missing, sugars build up and can cause developmental delays. This human trial was sponsored by Sangamo therapeutics, a biotech company based in Richmond, California. The company then inserts a replacement copy of the gene, using gene editing to snip the DNA helix of liver cells in a specific place near the promoter or on-off switch for the gene related to the albumin protein. The cells repaired the damage by inserting the DNA for the new gene, supplied by the researchers along with the DNA scissors of the gene editor, and the gene activity is then controlled by the powerful albumin promoter. The idea is to turn these modified liver cells into a factory for making the enzyme missing in the Hunter syndrome. On the other hand, other research works assess their effectiveness while many patents were in progress. Hence, the theme comprises multidisciplinary fields. Therefore, one of the main issues being discussed is related to the development of clinically viable delivery methods as one of the greatest challenges in the therapeutic application of CRISPR/Cas9-mediated genome edition.

For these reasons, many new approaches are in progress to improve their delivery based on cargo nanoarchitectures, such as thermo-triggered release of CRISPR-Cas9 system by laser excitation based on lipid-encapsulated gold nanoparticles for tumor therapy [39]. In order to do that, Cas9-sgPlk-1 plasmids (CP) were condensed on TAT peptide-modified Au nanoparticles (AuNPs/CP, ACP) *via* electrostatic interactions, and coated lipids (DOTAP, DOPE, cholesterol, PEG2000-DSPE) on the ACP to form lipid encapsulated, AuNPs-condensed CP (LACP). Thus, LACP could enter the tumor cells and release CP into the cytosol by the laser-triggered thermo-effects of the AuNPs; the CP could enterthe nuclei by TAT guidance, enabling effective knock-outs of target gene (Plk-1) of tumor (melanoma) and inhibition of the tumor both *in vitro* and *in vivo*.

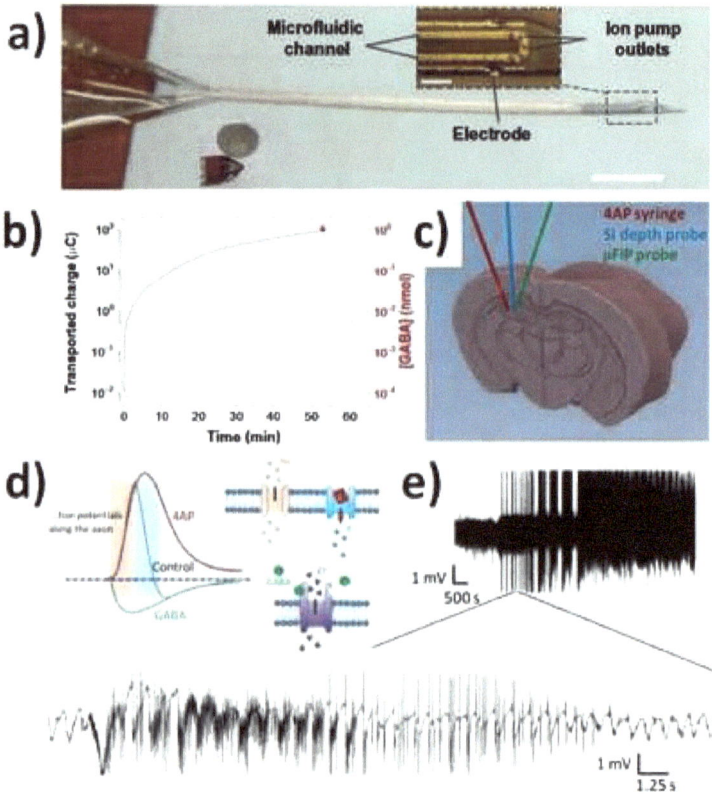

Fig. (4). Overview of the µFIP probe. **a)** Implanted end of the device (inset scale bar, 100 µm; outside scale bar, 1 mm). **b)** Net transported charge across the ion bridge when actively pumping GABA at 1 V (line, left axis), [GABA] passively diffused out of the device when no voltage was applied (open symbols, right axis), and [GABA] actively pumped out of the device at 1 V (closed symbols, right axis). **c)** Scheme showing placement of syringe for 4AP injection, Si depth probe and the µFIP probe in the hippocampus. **d)** Conceptual illustration showing a proposed effect of 4AP on K^+ channels and action potentials along with the analogous effects of GABA. **e)** Representative recording of intense seizure-like events (SLEs) following injection of 4AP at two different time scales [32].

Similarly, modified gold cores allowed nanoparticle delivery of CRISPR into the brain of a mouse model for specific syndrome from exaggerated repetitive behaviours [40]. The researchers injected CRISPR-gold into two brain areas in mice and found that the system edited genes in several major cell types. It should also be noted that the development of lipid NPs enabled the delivery of the CRISPR/Cas9 enzymatic gen editor for mouse transthyretin (Ttr) gene in the liver [41], with >97% reduction in protein levels that persisted for unless 12 months. These types of studies were conducted with patents from important companies such as Merck, considering critics from other research works and ethical discussions.

There are other gene delivery pathways and gene edition strategies based on the incorporation of virus and gene editing of CCR5 in autologous CD4 T cells [42] of people infected with HIV [43]. The CCR5 is the major co-receptor for human immunodeficiency virus (HIV). Here, research tried to investigate whether site-specific modification of the gene ("gene editing"). In this case, the infusion of the used autologous CD4 T cells were with the CCR5 gene rendered permanently dysfunctional by a zinc-finger nuclease (ZFN) . In this manner, from human trials developed from human blood, even if decreased levels of HIV DNA were recorded in most patients, some adverse events were associated with infusion of the ZFN-modified autologous CD4 T cells; thus, the theme still being in study. Moreover, a recent study in human trials related to gene therapy was reported in patients with transfusion-dependent β-Thalassemia [44], where a diminished media annualized transfusion volume of 73% was recorded with three cases of discontinued red cell transfusion from a total of 13 patients tested. Finally, we should mention the new approaches in progress in the frontiers of genomic level.

CONCLUDING REMARKS

Personalized nanomedicine demonstrated to be a high-impact research field that derived, in some cases, in many patents and legal debates. These themes, in addition to big data collection, privacy issues and online telemedicine, are ongoing topics of discussion for the future of medicine. It should be highlighted how, from the simple control of the nanoscales and insights gained from molecular biology and genetics, a wide range of technological developments has taken place, including miniaturized devices and instrumentations.

REFERENCES

[1]   D. Darvill, A. Centeno, and F. Xie, "Plasmonic fluorescence enhancement by metalnanostructures: Shaping the future of bionanotechnology", , vol. 38, pp. 1-4, 2013.

[2]   K. Golberg, A. Elbaz, R. McNeil, A. Kushmaro, C.D. Geddes, and R.S. Marks, "Increased bioassay sensitivity of bioactive molecule discovery using metal-enhanced bioluminescence", *J. Nanopart. Res.,* vol. 16, no. 2770, pp. 1-14, 2014.
        [http://dx.doi.org/10.1007/s11051-014-2770-y]

[3]   D. Brouard, M.L. Viger, A.G. Bracamonte, and D. Boudreau, "Label-free biosensing based on multilayer fluorescent nanocomposites and a cationic polymeric transducer", *ACS Nano,* vol. 5, no. 3, pp. 1888-1896, 2011.
        [http://dx.doi.org/10.1021/nn102776m] [PMID: 21344882]

[4]   D. Brouard, O. Ratelle, A.G. Bracamonte, M. St-Louis, and D. Boudreau, "Direct molecular detection of SRY gene from unamplified genomic DNA by metal enhanced fluorescence and FRET", *Anal. Methods,* vol. 5, pp. 6896-6899, 2013.
        [http://dx.doi.org/10.1039/c3ay41428k]

[5]   D. Brouard, O. Ratelle, J. Perreault, D. Boudreau, and M. St-Louis, "PCR-free blood group genotyping using a nanobiosensor", *Vox Sang.,* vol. 108, no. 2, pp. 197-204, 2015.
        [http://dx.doi.org/10.1111/vox.12207] [PMID: 25469570]

[6]   Y. Zhao, R.K. Kankala, S-B. Wang, and A-Z. Chen, "Multi-organs-on-chips: Towards long-term biomedical investigations", *Molecules,* vol. 24, no. 4, pp. 1-22, 2019.
[http://dx.doi.org/10.3390/molecules24040675] [PMID: 30769788]

[7]   C. Le Tourneau, E. Borcoman, and M. Kamal, "Molecular profiling in precision medicine oncology, Nature Medicine", *News Views,* pp. 1-2, 2019.

[8]   J. Rodon, J-C. Soria, R. Berger, W.H. Miller, E. Rubin, A. Kugel, A. Tsimberidou, P. Saintigny, A. Ackerstein, I. Braña, Y. Loriot, M. Afshar, V. Miller, F. Wunder, C. Bresson, J-F. Martini, J. Raynaud, J. Mendelsohn, G. Batist, A. Onn, J. Tabernero, R.L. Schilsky, V. Lazar, J.J. Lee, and R. Kurzrock, "Genomic and transcriptomic profiling expands precision cancer medicine: the WINTHER trial", *Nat. Med.,* vol. 25, no. 5, pp. 751-758, 2019.
[http://dx.doi.org/10.1038/s41591-019-0424-4] [PMID: 31011205]

[9]   R. Bumgarner, "DNA microarrays: types, applications and their future", *Curr Protoc Mol Biol.,* vol. 22, no. 22.1, pp. 1-17, 2013.

[10]   C. O'Connor, "Fluorescence in situ hybridization (FISH)", *Nature Education,* vol. 1, no. 1, p. 171, 2008.

[11]   G.E. Palomaki, E.M. Kloza, G.M. Lambert-Messerlian, J.E. Haddow, L.M. Neveux, M. Ehrich, D. van den Boom, A.T. Bombard, C. Deciu, W.W. Grody, S.F. Nelson, and J.A. Canick, "DNA sequencing of maternal plasma to detect Down syndrome: an international clinical validation study", *Genet. Med.,* vol. 13, no. 11, pp. 913-920, 2011.
[http://dx.doi.org/10.1097/GIM.0b013e3182368a0e] [PMID: 22005709]

[12]   M. Reyes, D. Vickers, K. Billman, T. Eisenhaure, and P. Hoover, "Multiplexed enrichment and genomic profiling of peripheral blood cells reveal subset-specific immune signatures", *Sci. Adv,* vol. 5, pp. 1-10, 2019.
[PMID: eaau9223]

[13]   A.R. Warden, W. Liu, H. Chen, and X. Ding, "Portable infrared isothermal PCR platform for multiple sexually transmitted diseases strand detection", *Anal. Chem.,* vol. 90, no. 20, pp. 11760-11763, 2018.
[http://dx.doi.org/10.1021/acs.analchem.8b03507] [PMID: 30216046]

[14]   S. Chong, C. Dugast-Darzacq, Z. Liu, P. Dong, G. M. Dailey, C. Cattoglio, A. Heckert, S. Banala, L. Lavis, X. Darzacq, and R. Tjian, "Imaging dynamic and selective low-complexity domain interactions that control gene transcription", *Science,* vol. 361, no. 6400, pp. 1-2, 2018.
[PMID: eaar2555]

[15]   L. Mo, Z. Zhao, X. Hu, X. Yu, Y. Peng, H. Liu, M. Xiong, T. Fu, Y. Jiang, X. Zhang, and W. Tan, "Smart nanodrug with nuclear localization sequences in the presence of MMP-2 to overcome biobarriers and drug resistance", *Chemistry,* vol. 25, no. 8, pp. 1895-1900, 2019.
[http://dx.doi.org/10.1002/chem.201805107] [PMID: 30681205]

[16]   C. Wong, T. Stylianopoulos, J. Cui, J. Martin, V.P. Chauhan, W. Jiang, Z. Popovic, R.K. Jain, M.G. Bawendi, and D. Fukumura, "Multistage nanoparticle delivery system for deep penetration into tumor tissue", *Proc. Natl. Acad. Sci. USA,* vol. 108, no. 6, pp. 2426-2431, 2011.
[http://dx.doi.org/10.1073/pnas.1018382108] [PMID: 21245339]

[17]   R, Xu, G. Zhang, J. Mai, X. Dng, V. Segura-Ibarra, S. Wu, J. Shen, H. Liu, Z. Hu, L. Chen, Y. Huang, E. Koay, Y. Huang, J. Liu, J. E. Ensor, E. Balnco, x. Liu, M. Ferrari, and H. Shen, "An injectable nanoparticle generator enhances delivery of cancer therapeutics", *Nat. Biotechnol.,* vol. 34, pp. 414-418, 2016.

[18]   D. Gontero, M. Lessard-Viger, D. Brouard, A.G. Bracamonte, D. Boudreau, and A.V. Veglia, "Smart Multifunctional Nanoparticles design as Sensors and Drug delivery systems based on Supramolecular chemistry", *Microchem. J.,* vol. 130, pp. 316-328, 2017.
[http://dx.doi.org/10.1016/j.microc.2016.10.007]

[19]   *J. Polym. Sci. A Polym. Chem.,* vol. 38, pp. 1673-1679, 2000.

[http://dx.doi.org/10.1002/(SICI)1099-0518(20000501)38:9<1673::AID-POLA33>3.0.CO;2-T]

[20] M.L. Hans, and A.M. Lowman, *Curr. Opin. Solid State Mater. Sci.,* vol. 6, pp. 319-327, 2002.
[http://dx.doi.org/10.1016/S1359-0286(02)00117-1]

[21] S.I. Moon, C.W. Lee, M. Miyamoto, Y. Kimura, and R.A. Jain, *Biomaterials,* vol. 21, pp. 2475-2490, 2000.
[http://dx.doi.org/10.1016/S0142-9612(00)00115-0] [PMID: 11055295]

[22] B. Semete, L. Booysen, Y. Lemmer, L. Kalombo, L. Katata, J. Verschoor, and H.S. Swai, "Nanomedicine: Nanotech", *Biol. Med. (Aligarh),* vol. 6, pp. 662-671, 2010.

[23] L. Wang, K.G. Neoh, E.T. Kang, B. Shuter, and S.C. Wang, "Biodegradable magnetic-fluorescent magnetite/poly(dl-lactic acid-co-alpha,beta-malic acid) composite nanoparticles for stem cell labeling", *Biomaterials,* vol. 31, no. 13, pp. 3502-3511, 2010.
[http://dx.doi.org/10.1016/j.biomaterials.2010.01.081] [PMID: 20144844]

[24] Y. Liu, and A. Aguzzi, "Immunotherapy for neurodegeneration?", *Science,* vol. 364, no. 6436, pp. 130-131, 2019.
[PMID: 30975878]

[25] L. Voorwerk, M. Slagter, H.M. Horlings, K. Sikorska, K.K. van de Vijver, M. de Maaker, I. Nederlof, R.J.C. Kluin, S. Warren, S. Ong, T.G. Wiersma, N.S. Russell, F. Lalezari, P.C. Schouten, N.A.M. Bakker, S.L.C. Ketelaars, D. Peters, C.A.H. Lange, E. van Werkhoven, H. van Tinteren, I.A.M. Mandjes, I. Kemper, S. Onderwater, M. Chalabi, S. Wilgenhof, J.B.A.G. Haanen, R. Salgado, K.E. de Visser, G.S. Sonke, L.F.A. Wessel, S.C. Linn, T.N. Schumacher, C.U. Blank, and M. Kok, "Immune induction strategies in metastatic triple-negative breast cancer to enhance the sensitivity to PD-1 blockade: the TONIC trial", *Nat. Med.,* pp. 1-27, 2019.

[26] S. Tran, P-J. DeGiovanni, B. Piel, and P. Rai, "Cancer nanomedicine: a review of recent success in drug delivery", *Clin. Transl. Med.,* vol. 6, no. 1, p. 44, 2017.
[http://dx.doi.org/10.1186/s40169-017-0175-0] [PMID: 29230567]

[27] O. F. Khan, and P. S. Kowalski, " Endothelial siRNA delivery in nonhuman primates using ionizable low–molecular weight polymeric nanoparticles", *Sci. Adv,* vol. 4, no. , pp. 1-10, 2018.
[PMID: eaar8409]

[28] J.M. Wolfe, C.M. Fadzen, R.L. Holden, M. Yao, G.J. Hanson, and B.L. Pentelute, "Perfluoroaryl bicyclic cell-penetrating peptides for delivery of antisense oligonucleotides", *Angew. Chem. Int. Ed. Engl.,* vol. 57, no. 17, pp. 4756-4759, 2018.
[http://dx.doi.org/10.1002/anie.201801167] [PMID: 29479836]

[29] M.E. Davis, J.E. Zuckerman, C.H. Choi, D. Seligson, A. Tolcher, C.A. Alabi, Y. Yen, J.D. Heidel, A. Ribas, and A. Ribas, "Evidence of RNAi in humans from systemically administered siRNA via targeted nanoparticles", *Nature,* vol. 464, no. 7291, pp. 1067-1070, 2010.
[http://dx.doi.org/10.1038/nature08956] [PMID: 20305636]

[30] Z. Zawada, A. Tatar, P. Mocilac, M. Buděšínský, and T. Kraus, "Transport of nucleoside triphosphates into cells by artificial molecular transporters", *Angew. Chem. Int. Ed. Engl.,* vol. 57, no. 31, pp. 9891-9895, 2018.
[http://dx.doi.org/10.1002/anie.201801306] [PMID: 29578619]

[31] E.I. Mancera-Andrade, A. Parsaeimehr, and A. Arevalo-Gallegos, G. Ascencio- Favela, and R. Parra-Saldiva, "Microfluidics technology for drug delivery: a review, frontiers in bioscience", *Elite,* vol. 10, pp. 74-91, 2018.

[32] C.M. Proctor, A. Slézia, A. Kaszas, A. Ghestem, I. Del Agua, A.M. Pappa, C. Bernard, A. Williamson, and G.G. Malliaras, "Electrophoretic drug delivery for seizure control", *Sci. Adv.,* vol. 4, no. 8, 2018.eaau1291
[http://dx.doi.org/10.1126/sciadv.aau1291] [PMID: 30167463]

[33] H. Takehara, A. Nagaoka, J. Noguchi, T. Akagi, H. Kasai, and T. Ichiki, "Lab-on-a-brain: implantable

micro-optical fluidic devices for neural cell analysis *in vivo*", *Sci. Rep.,* vol. 4, no. 6721, p. 6721, 2014.
[PMID: 25335545]

[34]   E.H. Chang, J.B. Harford, M.A.W. Eaton, P.M. Boisseau, A. Dube, R. Hayeshi, H. Swai, and D.S.
Lee, "Nanomedicine: Past, present and future - A global perspective", *Biochem. Biophys. Res.
Commun.,* vol. 468, no. 3, pp. 511-517, 2015.
[http://dx.doi.org/10.1016/j.bbrc.2015.10.136] [PMID: 26518648]

[35]   P. Liang, Y. Xu, X. Zhang, C. Ding, R. Huang, Z. Zhang, J. Lv, X. Xie, Y. Chen, Y. Li, Y. Sun, Y.
Bai, Z. Songyang, W. Ma, C. Zhou, and J. Huang, "CRISPR/Cas9-mediated gene editing in human
tripronuclear zygotes", *Protein Cell,* vol. 6, no. 5, pp. 363-372, 2015.
[http://dx.doi.org/10.1007/s13238-015-0153-5] [PMID: 25894090]

[36]   J. Cohen, "In dogs, CRISPR fixes a muscular dystrophy", *Science,* vol. 361, no. 6405, pp. 835-839,
2018.
[http://dx.doi.org/10.1126/science.361.6405.835] [PMID: 30166469]

[37]   E. Pennisi, "Transgenic animals. Editing of targeted genes proved possible in monkeys", *Science,* vol.
343, no. 6170, pp. 476-477, 2014.
[http://dx.doi.org/10.1126/science.343.6170.476] [PMID: 24482459]

[38]   J. Kaiser, *A human has been injected with gene-editing tools to cure his disabling disease. Here's what
you need to know, Science News.* AAAS, 2017, pp. 1-2.

[39]   P. Wang, L. Zhang, W. Zheng, L. Cong, Z. Guo, Y. Xie, L. Wang, R. Tang, Q. Feng, Y. Hamada, K.
Gonda, Z. Hu, X. Wu, and X. Jiang, "Thermo-triggered Release of CRISPR-Cas9 system by lipid-
encapsulated gold nanoparticles for tumor therapy", *Angew. Chem. Int. Ed. Engl.,* vol. 57, no. 6, pp.
1491-1496, 2018.
[http://dx.doi.org/10.1002/anie.201708689] [PMID: 29282854]

[40]   B. Lee, K. Lee, S. Panda, R. Gonzales-Rojas, A. Chong, V. Bugay, H.M. Park, R. Brenner, N. Murthy,
and H.Y. Lee, "Nanoparticle delivery of CRISPR into the brain rescues a mouse model of fragile X
syndrome from exaggerated repetitive behaviours", *Nat. Biomed. Eng.,* vol. 2, no. 7, pp. 497-507,
2018.
[http://dx.doi.org/10.1038/s41551-018-0252-8] [PMID: 30948824]

[41]   J.D. Finn, A.R. Smith, M.C. Patel, L. Shaw, M.R. Youniss, J. van Heteren, T. Dirstine, C. Ciullo, R.
Lescarbeau, J. Seitzer, R.R. Shah, A. Shah, D. Ling, J. Growe, M. Pink, E. Rohde, K.M. Wood, W.E.
Salomon, W.F. Harrington, C. Dombrowski, W.R. Strapps, Y. Chang, and D.V. Morrissey, "A Single
Administration of CRISPR/Cas9 Lipid Nanoparticles Achieves Robust and Persistent In Vivo Genome
Editing", *Cell Rep.,* vol. 22, no. 9, pp. 2227-2235, 2018.
[http://dx.doi.org/10.1016/j.celrep.2018.02.014] [PMID: 29490262]

[42]   P. Tebas, D. Stein, G. Binder-Scholl, R. Mukherjee, T. Brady, T. Rebello, L. Humeau, M. Kalos, E.
Papasavvas, L.J. Montaner, D. Schullery, F. Shaheen, A.L. Brennan, Z. Zheng, J. Cotte, V.
Slepushkin, E. Veloso, A. Mackley, W.T. Hwang, F. Aberra, J. Zhan, J. Boyer, R.G. Collman, F.D.
Bushman, B.L. Levine, and C.H. June, "Antiviral effects of autologous CD4 T cells genetically
modified with a conditionally replicating lentiviral vector expressing long antisense to HIV", *Blood,*
vol. 121, no. 9, pp. 1524-1533, 2013.
[http://dx.doi.org/10.1182/blood-2012-07-447250] [PMID: 23264589]

[43]   P. Tebas, D. Stein, W.W. Tang, I. Frank, S.Q. Wang, G. Lee, S.K. Spratt, R.T. Surosky, M.A. Giedlin,
G. Nichol, M.C. Holmes, P.D. Gregory, D.G. Ando, M. Kalos, R.G. Collman, G. Binder-Scholl, G.
Plesa, W-T. Hwang, B.L. Levine, and C.H. June, "Gene editing of CCR5 in autologous CD4 T cells of
persons infected with HIV", *N. Engl. J. Med.,* vol. 370, no. 10, pp. 901-910, 2014.
[http://dx.doi.org/10.1056/NEJMoa1300662] [PMID: 24597865]

[44]   A.A. Thompson, M.C. Walters, J. Kwiatkowski, J.E.J. Rasko, J.A. Ribeil, S. Hongeng, E. Magrin, G.J.
Schiller, E. Payen, M. Semeraro, D. Moshous, F. Lefrere, H. Puy, P. Bourget, A. Magnani, L.
Caccavelli, J.S. Diana, F. Suarez, F. Monpoux, V. Brousse, C. Poirot, C. Brouzes, J.F. Meritet, C.
Pondarré, Y. Beuzard, S. Chrétien, T. Lefebvre, D.T. Teachey, U. Anurathapan, P.J. Ho, C. von Kalle,

M. Kletzel, E. Vichinsky, S. Soni, G. Veres, O. Negre, R.W. Ross, D. Davidson, A. Petrusich, L. Sandler, M. Asmal, O. Hermine, M. De Montalembert, S. Hacein-Bey-Abina, S. Blanche, P. Leboulch, and M. Cavazzana, "Gene therapy in patients with transfusion-dependent β-thalassemia", *N. Engl. J. Med.,* vol. 378, no. 16, pp. 1479-1493, 2018.
[http://dx.doi.org/10.1056/NEJMoa1705342] [PMID: 29669226]

CHAPTER 15

State-of-the-Art Technology

All these sections have discussed a variety of themes ranging from the control of the nanoscale by the design of different nanoarchitectures with variable methodologies to their incorporate for the development of nano-, and microdevices for specific applications. For these reasons, future perspectives involve many fields and challenges to face. However, we could still identify challenges in progress and discuss new ones.

In this way, from synthetic methodologies in colloidal dispersions even, many synthetic pathways are reported of many materials in the literature as well as their incorporation into nanoparticles and microparticles as tools within life sciences fabricated from the most important companies in the market; a small fraction from a huge number of possibilities was developed. Thus, there are still synthetic methodologies that have not yet been devised for multifunctional platforms at different scale levels. These particles could be considered as miniaturized devices for required applications to achieve functionalization. Steps should be taken for design, synthesis and characterization to fabricate functional devices on the particle. Some types of particles of interest include the control of size and shape in different types of particles, such as hybrid particles, multi-layered and multi-core-shell particles where inorganic materials and organic composites are involved, Janus particles where chemical surface modifications assume relevance just as for particle functionalization. Definitely, these themes form part of different applications. The importance of developments in areas such as signal transduction and amplification, linked to the design of light-emitting devices incorporating non-classical light generation, conductive particles, wires and their inclusion in devices, their application in life sciences such as lab-on particles in genomics and nanomedicine and multi-modal imaging has to be noted [1].

Moreover, the miniaturized surfaces of varying sizes could be added to accurately designed devices by lithography technique based on multi-layered deposition of inorganic and organic masks. In this way, different patterned guides could be developed for signal transduction as well as particle deposition, confinement and flow. Here, from major research on metamaterials may derive the next highly technological materials, for instance, in Waveguiding approaches. The development and direct application of high-power irradiancy lasers may also be underlined for a controlled cutting, marking and designing, and their miniaturization for incorporation in miniaturized devices based on waveguides and micro- to nanofluidic systems, including surface modification, grating with varied size for enhanced interactions and generation of nanolasers for targeted molecular applications. Within this large field, numerous studies report the control and generation of classical and non-classical light based on hybrid nano-[2, 3] and micro-platforms [4], with characterization and evaluation of biocompatibility, where each part of the nanodevice takes on a vital role (Fig. **1**).

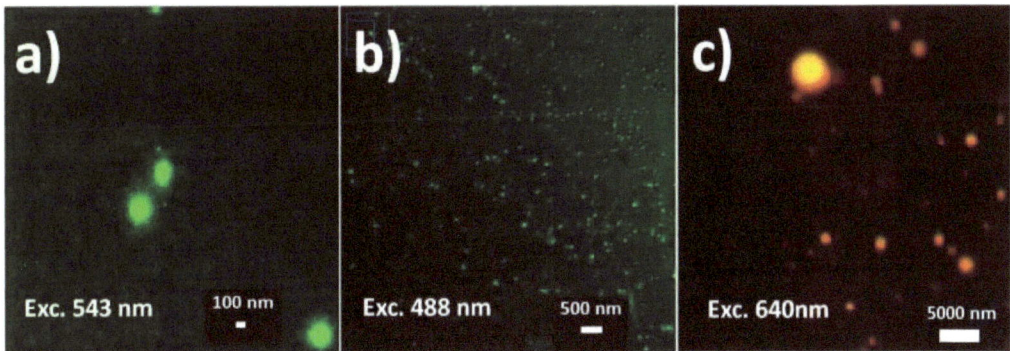

Fig. (1). Laser fluorescence microscopy imaging of nano- and micro-platforms at different excitation wavelengths: **a)** Ultraluminescent biocompatible gold core-shell nanoparticles of 50 nm average diameters based on metal enhanced fluorescence (**MEF**). Laser excitation= 543.0 nm. Reprinted with permission from D. Boudreau – G. Bracamonte *et al*. Copyright 2018 Journal of Nanophotonics [1]. **b)** Enhanced luminescent polymeric nanoplatforms based on fluorescence resonance energy transfer (**FRET**). Laser excitation= 488.0 nm. Reprinted with permission from V. Ame – G. Bracamonte *et al*. Copyright 2019 Ed. Académica Española, OmniScriptum GmbH [2]. **c)** Luminescent cargo-loaded hybrid vesicles. Laser excitation= 640.0 nm [4].

To conclude, many of the last Nobel Prizes were awarded to research and technological applications. For example, it could be mentioned that the 2010 Nobel Prize in Physics was given for goundbreaking experiments regarding the two-dimensional material graphene for its incorporations within composite materials of electronic devices; while in 2014 the award in Chemistry was given for controlled light emission at single-molecule level for enhanced image resolution applications such as super-resolved fluorescence microscopy. Another 2016 award was granted in Chemistry for the design and synthesis of molecular machines. In 2017, the development of super-resolved cryo-electron microscopy for high resolution at the biomolecular level was also awarded a Nobel Prize in Chemistry. In 2018 an award was given in Chemistry to the directed evolution of enzymes and to the phage display of peptides and antibodies, with strong implications in immunochemistry and pharmaceutical industry. In 2018, the award was given to ground-breaking inventions in the field of laser physics and tools made of light, such as ultrashort high-intensity beams, known as chirped-pulse amplification, for high accurate resolution eye surgery applications. Finally, the Nobel Prize in 2018 was awarded for physiology or medicine for the discovery of cancer therapy by inhibition of negative immune regulation, influencing new targeted drugs and immune cancer therapies.

So, Fundamental Research focused on objectives based on high impact social needs is in rapid progress. In the precedent chapters, it was intended to motivate the readers to participate in different Research fields involucrated from acquiring the knowledge, discover new challenges and needs, and to develop solutions.

REFERENCES

[1]   H. Kim, H. Lee, H. Moon, J. Kang, Y. Jang, D. Kim, J. Kim, E. Huynh, G. Zheng, H. Kim, and J. Ho Chang, "Resonance-Based Frequency-Selective Amplification for Increased Photoacoustic Imaging Sensitivity", *ACS Photonics,* vol. 692, pp. 268-2276, 2019.
       [http://dx.doi.org/10.1021/acsphotonics.9b00576]

[2]   D. Gontero, A. V. Veglia, D. Boudreau, and A. G. Bracamonte, Ultraluminescent gold Core@shell nanoparticles applied to individual bacterial detection based on Metal-Enhanced Fluorescence Nanoimaging, J. of Nanophotonics. Special issue Nanoplasmonics for Biosensing, Enhanced Light-Matter Interaction, and Spectral Engineering, 12, 1, 012505 (2018) 1-12.

[3]   A. G. Bracamonte, C. I. Salinas, and M. V. Ame, Enhanced luminescent nanoplatforms based on FRET. Biophotonics applications", Ed. Académica Española: OmniScriptum GmbH & Co. KG, ISBN 978-613-9-44056-6 (2019).

[4]   A.G. Bracamonte, D. Boudreau, W. Landis, and N. Sahai, From Origin of life to Synthetic Biology developments and Biotechnological applications, Bitácora digital Journal. Open call, 9º Ed., Faculty of Chem. Sc. (UNC), 1, 9 (2018) ISNN: 2344-9144.

SUBJECT INDEX

www.ingramcontent.com/pod-product-compliance
Lightning Source LLC
Chambersburg PA
CBHW041710210326
41598CB00007B/600